Praise for
The Glucose Revolution and The Glucose Revolution Pocket Guides

■

"Forget *Sugar Busters*. Forget *The Zone*. If you want the real scoop on how carbohydrates and sugar affect your body, read this book by the world's leading researchers on the subject. It's the authoritative, last word on choosing foods to control your blood sugar."
—JEAN CARPER, best-selling author of *Miracle Cures, Stop Aging Now!* and *Food: Your Miracle Medicine*

■

"The concept of the glycemic index has been distorted and bastardized by popular writers and diet gurus. Here, at last, is a book that explains what we know about the glycemic index and its importance in designing a diet for optimum health. Carbohydrates are not all bad. Read the good news about pasta and even—believe it or not—sugar!"
—ANDREW WEIL, M.D., University of Arizona College of Medicine, author of *Spontaneous Healing* and *8 Weeks to Optimum Health*

■

"Here is at last a book explaining the importance of taking into consideration the glycemic index of foods for overall health, athletic performance, and in reducing the risk of heart disease and diabetes. The book clearly explains that there are different kinds of carbohydrates that work in different ways and why a universal recommendation to 'increase the carbohydrate content of your diet' is plainly simple and scientifically inaccurate. Everyone should put the glycemic index approach into practice."

—ARTEMIS P. SIMOPOULOS, M.D., senior author of *The Omega Diet* and *The Healing Diet* and President, The Center for Genetics, Nutrition and Health, Washington, D.C.

■

"*The Glucose Revolution* is nutrition science for the 21st century. Clearly written, it gives the scientific rationale for why all carbohydrates are not created equal. It is a practical guide for both professionals and patients. The food suggestions and recipes are exciting and tasty."

—RICHARD N. PODELL, M.D., M.P.H., Clinical Professor, Department of Family Medicine, UMDNJ–Robert Wood Johnson Medical School, and co-author of *The G-Index Diet: The Missing Link That Makes Permanent Weight Loss Possible*

■

"Although the jury is still out on the utility of the glycemic index, many of the curious will benefit from a careful reading of this book, and some will find that the glycemic index is particularly helpful for them. Everyone can enjoy the recipes, some of which are to die for!"

—JOHANNA DWYER, D. Sc., R.D., editor, *Nutrition Today*

The Glucose Revolution Pocket Guide to
SUGAR AND ENERGY

OTHER *GLUCOSE REVOLUTION* TITLES

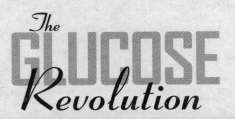

The GLUCOSE Revolution

POCKET GUIDE TO
SUGAR AND ENERGY

JENNIE BRAND-MILLER, PH.D.

KAYE FOSTER-POWELL, M. NUTR. & DIET.

THOMAS M.S. WOLEVER, M.D., PH.D.

ADAPTED BY

JOHANNA BURANI, M.S., R.D., C.D.E.,

AND LINDA RAO, M.ED.

■

MARLOWE & COMPANY
NEW YORK

Published by
Marlowe & Company
841 Broadway, 4th Floor
New York, NY 10003

The information in this book is intended to help readers make informed decisions about their health and the health of their loved ones. It is not intended to be a substitute for treatment by or the advice and care of a professional health care provider. While the authors and publisher have endeavored to ensure that the information is accurate and up to date, they are not responsible for adverse effects or consequences sustained by any person using this book.

First published in Australia in 1998 in somewhat different form under the title *Pocket Guide to the G.I. Factor and Sugar and Energy* by Hodder Headline Australia Pty Limited.

This edition is published by arrangement with Hodder Headline Australia Pty Limited.

Library of Congress Cataloging-in-Publication Data

Brand-Miller, Janette, 1952-
    The glucose revolution pocket guide to sugar and energy / by Jennie Brand-Miller, Kaye Foster-Powell, and Thomas M.S. Wolever.
        p.   cm.
    ISBN 1-56924-641-6
    1. Sugar—Health aspects.   2. Glycemic index.   3. Blood sugar.
4. Energy metabolism.   I. Title: Glucose revolution.
II. Foster-Powell, Kaye.   III. Wolever, Thomas M.S.   IV. Title.

QP702.S8 B73 2000
612.3'96—dc21
                                                                    00-021902

9 8 7 6 5 4 3 2 1

Designed by Pauline Neuwirth, Neuwirth & Associates, Inc.
Distributed by Publishers Group West
Manufactured in the United States of America

CONTENTS

PREFACE

The Glucose Revolution is the definitive, all-in-one guide to the glycemic index. Now we have written this pocket guide to show you how the glycemic index (G.I.) relates to sugar and its effects on the body. As we explain in *The Glucose Revolution*, the glycemic index:

- is a proven guide to the true physiological effects foods—especially carbohydrates—have on blood sugar levels;
- provides an easy and effective way to eat a healthy diet and control fluctuations in blood sugar.

This book offers more in-depth information about how sugar relates to the glycemic index than we had room to include in *The Glucose Revolution*. Much new information appears in this book that is not in *The Glucose Revolution*, including sample menus and the questions people most frequently ask about sugar.

This book has been written to be read alongside *The Glucose Revolution*, so in the event you haven't already consulted that book, please be sure to do so, for a more comprehensive discussion of the glycemic index and all its uses.

Chapter 1

INTRODUCTION

---

*M*any people today are convinced that sugar is a real "no-no"—one of the evils of modern diets and responsible (virtually on its own!) for a multitude of human diseases. Others are not quite so negative, but still regard sugar as one of those things people can easily do without—because it's simply not necessary and you benefit by avoiding it.

These messages are what many doctors, dentists, nutritionists and health authorities have preached for many years, and some still hold fast to these opinions despite the scientific evidence we now have. Their negative views of sugar stem from studies in the 1960s and 1970s that associated sugar with "empty calories," rapid weight gain (in rats!) and dental cavities. Nutrition science and public health have progressed markedly since then, but unfortunately some of the mud still sticks.

For the past twenty years, sugar has been the subject of close scientific scrutiny worldwide and the evidence from hundreds of studies clearly indicates that sugar is not the villain it was once thought to be. In the opinion of the world's leading nutrition authorities including the World Health Organization (WHO) and the Food and Agriculture Organization of the United Nations (FAO), reasonable intake of sugar-rich foods can provide for a palatable and nutritious diet.

If we look at the recent scientific evidence objectively, the findings suggest that avoiding sugar may do you more harm than good. There are undesirable aspects of diets that are low in sugars. The vast array of sugar-free and "no added sugar" foods on supermarket shelves has not solved the problem of overweight and obesity. In fact, it could be said that they have exacerbated the problem.

In this book we take a look at the scientifically proven breakthroughs about sugar and energy; dispel some common myths; reveal why it's high time to get rid of the guilt; and tell you what you really need to know about sugar, your health and blood sugar control, weight loss, dental cavities and behavior and mental performance.

Our intention is not to encourage an excessive amount of sugar. Excess of anything is not a good idea! We want you to feel that a reasonable quantity of sugar—about 10 to 12 percent of total calories per day—can be part of a well-balanced diet. Unfortunately, this amount is less than we currently eat in the United States. Luckily, this book tells you how to make this lower amount a reality by offering sample menus for adults, children and people with diabetes.

WHAT WE MEAN BY ENERGY

In a nutritional sense, "energy" equals the calories that become available when a food is digested and metabolized within the body. The energy content of a food provides a measure of that food's capacity to provide our fuel requirements. Some foods provide more energy than others. High fat foods have the greatest energy content: 1 gram of fat breaks down into 9 calories, while 1 gram of carbohydrate (sugar) or protein provides less than half that, or just 4 calories.

Chapter 2

THE GLYCEMIC INDEX: SOME BACKGROUND

HOW THE MILLS CHANGED EVERYTHING
HOW THE GLYCEMIC INDEX CAME TO BE
WHAT IS THE GLYCEMIC INDEX?
THE GLYCEMIC INDEX MADE SIMPLE
MEASURING THE GLYCEMIC INDEX

For the past 10,000 years, our ancestors survived on a high carbohydrate and low fat diet. They ate their carbohydrates in the form of beans, vegetables and whole cereal grains, and got their sugars from fibrous fruits and berries. Food preparation was a simple process: They ground food between stones and cooked it over the heat of an open fire. The result? All of their food was digested and absorbed slowly, which raised their blood sugar levels more slowly and over a longer period of time.

This diet was ideal for their bodies because it provided slow release energy that helped to delay hunger pangs and provided fuel for working muscles long after the meal was eaten. The slow rise in blood sugar was also kind to the pancreas, the organ that produces insulin.

HOW THE MILLS CHANGED EVERYTHING

As time passed, flours were ground more and more finely and bran was separated completely from the white flour. With the advent of high speed roller mills in the nineteenth century, it was possible to produce white flour so fine that it resembled talcum powder in appearance and texture. These fine white flours have always been highly prized because they make soft bread and light, airy sponge cakes. As incomes grew, people pushed their peas and beans aside and started eating more meat. As a consequence, the composition of the average diet changed, in that we began to eat more fat and because the type of carbohydrate in our diet changed, it became more quickly digested and absorbed. Something we didn't expect happened, too: The blood sugar rise after a meal was higher and more prolonged, stimulating the pancreas to produce more insulin.

THE PANCREAS PRODUCES INSULIN

The pancreas is a vital organ near the stomach, and its main job is to produce the hormone insulin. Carbohydrate stimulates the secretion of insulin more than any other component of food. The slow absorption of the carbohydrate in our food means that the pancreas doesn't have to work so hard and needs to produce less insulin. If the pancreas is overstimulated over a long period of time, it may become "exhausted" and type 2 diabetes can develop in genetically susceptible people. Even without diabetes, high insulin levels are undesirable because they increase the risk of heart disease.

Unfortunately, over time, we have begun to eat more "refined" foods and fewer "whole" foods. This new way of eating has brought with it higher blood sugar levels after a meal and higher insulin responses, as well. Though our bodies do need insulin for carbohydrate metabolism, high levels of the hormone have a profound effect on the development of many diseases. In fact, medical experts now believe that high insulin levels are one of the key factors responsible for heart disease and hypertension. Insulin influences the way we metabolize foods, determining whether we burn fat or carbohydrate to meet our energy needs and ultimately determining whether we store fat in our bodies.

HOW THE GLYCEMIC INDEX CAME TO BE

The glycemic index concept was first developed in 1981 by a team of scientists led by Dr. David Jenkins, a professor of nutrition at the University of Toronto, Canada, to help determine which foods were best for people with diabetes. At that time, the diet for people with diabetes was based on a system of carbohydrate exchanges or portions, which was complicated and not very logical. The carbohydrate exchange system assumed that all starchy foods produce the same effect on blood sugar levels even though some earlier studies had already proven this was not correct. Jenkins was one of the first researchers to question this assumption and to investigate how real foods behave in the bodies of real people.

Jenkins's approach attracted a great deal of attention because it was so logical and systematic. He and his colleagues had tested a large number of common foods, and some of their results were surprising. Ice cream, for example, despite its sugar content, had much less effect on blood sugar than some ordinary breads. Over the next 15 years medical researchers and scientists around the world, including the authors of this book, tested the effect of many foods on blood sugar levels and developed a new concept of classifying carbohydrates based on their glycemic index.

WHAT IS THE GLYCEMIC INDEX?

The glycemic index of foods is simply a ranking of foods based on their immediate effect on blood sugar levels. To make a fair comparison, all foods are compared with a reference food such as pure glucose and are tested in equivalent carbohydrate amounts.

Originally, research into the glycemic index of foods was inspired by the desire to identify the best foods for people with diabetes. But scientists are now discovering that G.I. values have implications for everyone.

Today we know the glycemic index of hundreds of different food items—both generic and name-brand—that have been tested following a standardized testing method. The tables in Chapter 17 on pages 82 to 101 give the glycemic index of a range of common foods, including many tested at the University of Toronto and the University of Sydney.

THE GLYCEMIC INDEX MADE SIMPLE

Carbohydrate foods that break down quickly during digestion have the highest G.I. values. The blood glucose, or sugar, response is fast and high. In other words the glucose in the bloodstream increases rapidly. Conversely, carbohydrates that break down slowly, releasing glucose gradually into the bloodstream, have low G.I. values. An analogy might be the popular fable of the tortoise and the hare. The hare, just like high G.I. foods, speeds away full steam ahead but loses the race to the tortoise with his slow and steady pace. Similarly, slow and steady low G.I. foods produce a smooth blood sugar curve without wild fluctuations.

For most people most of the time, the foods with a low glycemic index have advantages over those with high G.I. values. Figure 1 shows the effect of slow and fast carbohydrate on blood sugar levels(figure 1).

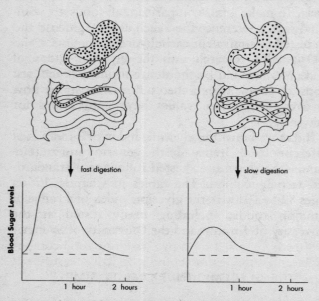

Figure 1. Slow and fast carbohydrate digestion and the consequent levels of sugar in the blood.

The substance that produces the greatest rise in blood sugar levels is pure glucose itself. All other foods have less effect when fed in equal amounts of carbohydrate. The glycemic index of pure glucose is set at 100, and every other food is ranked on a scale from 0 to 100 according to its actual effect on blood sugar levels.

The glycemic index of a food cannot be predicted from its composition or the glycemic index of related foods. To test the glycemic index, you need real people and real foods. We describe how the glycemic index of a food is measured below. There is no easy, inexpensive substitute test. Scientists always follow standardized methods so that results from one group of people can be directly compared with those of another group.

In total, 8 to 10 people need to be tested and the glycemic index of the food is the average value of the group. We know this average figure is reproducible and that a different group of volunteers will produce a similar result. Results obtained in a group of people with diabetes are comparable to those without diabetes.

The most important point to note is that all foods are tested in equivalent carbohydrate amounts. For example, 100 grams of bread (about 3½ slices of sandwich bread) is tested because this contains 50 grams of carbohydrate. Likewise, 60 grams of jelly beans (containing 50 grams of carbohydrate) is compared with the reference food. We know how much carbohydrate is in a food by consulting food composition tables, the manufacturer's data or measuring it ourselves in the laboratory.

■ ■ ■

■

THE GLYCEMIC INDEX IS A CLINICALLY PROVEN TOOL IN
ITS APPLICATIONS TO DIABETES, APPETITE CONTROL AND
REDUCING THE RISK OF HEART DISEASE.

■

MEASURING THE GLYCEMIC INDEX

Scientists use just six steps to determine the glycemic index of a food. Simple as this may sound, it's actually quite a time-consuming process. Here's how it works.

1. An amount of food containing 50 grams of carbohydrate is given to a volunteer to eat. For example, to test boiled spaghetti, the volunteer would be given 200 grams of spaghetti, which supplies 50 grams of carbohydrate (we work this out from food composition tables or by measuring the available carbohydrate)—50 grams of carbohydrate is equivalent to 3 tablespoons of pure glucose powder.

2. Over the next two hours (or three hours if the volunteer has diabetes), we take a sample of their blood every 15 minutes during the first hour and thereafter every 30 minutes. The blood sugar level of these blood samples is measured in the laboratory and recorded.

3. The blood sugar level is plotted on a graph and the area under the curve is calculated using a computer program (Figure 2).

4. The volunteer's response to spaghetti (or whatever food is being tested) is compared with his or her blood sugar response to 50 grams of pure glucose (the reference food).

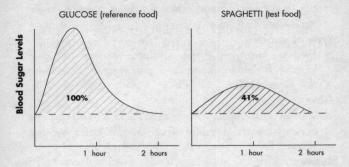

Figure 2. Measuring the glycemic index of a food. The effect of a food on blood sugar levels is calculated using the area under the curve (shaded area). The area under the curve after consumption of the test food is compared with the same area after the reference food (usually 50 grams of pure glucose or a 50 gram carbohydrate portion of white bread).

5. The reference food is tested on two or three separate occasions and an average value is calculated. This is done to reduce the effect of day-to-day variation in blood sugar responses.

6. The average glycemic index found in 8 to 10 people is the glycemic index of that food.

---

5 KEY FACTORS THAT INFLUENCE THE GLYCEMIC INDEX

Cooking methods

Cooking and processing increases the glycemic index of a food because it increases the amount of gelatinized starch in the food. Cornflakes is one example.

Physical form of the food

An intact fibrous coat, such as that on grains and legumes,

acts as a physical barrier and slows down digestion, lowering a food's G.I. value.

Type of starch

There are two types of starch in foods, amylose and amylopectin. The more amylose starch a food contains, the lower the glycemic index.

Fiber

Viscous, soluble fibers, such as those found in rolled oats and apples, slow down digestion and lower a food's glycemic index.

Sugar

The presence of sugar, as well as the type of sugar, will influence a food's glycemic index. Fruits with a low glycemic index, such as apples and oranges, are high in fructose.

Chapter 3

WHAT *EXACTLY* IS SUGAR?

HOW MUCH HONEY DID OUR ANCESTORS EAT?

ALL ABOUT ADDED SUGAR

LOW FAT DIETS AND SUGAR INTAKE

The term "sugar" means different things to different people and the terminology can be confusing. In this book, as in everyday language, "sugar" refers to refined cane sugar, unless otherwise indicated. Sugar from sugar cane is a major source of this sweetener in American diets. "Sucrose" is the scientific name for the substance that contributes most of the sweetness in our diet.

The white granular powder extracted from sugar cane that we put in sugar bowls, cakes, cookies, and ice cream is similar to the principal sugar—and source of sweetness—in fruit, which contains a mixture of glucose, fructose and sucrose. (The sugar in soft drinks comes from high fructose corn syrup, which is a mixture of glucose and fructose. In the body, though, this mixture behaves exactly like sucrose.)

Sucrose is chemically classified as a carbohydrate and a simple sugar. Specifically, it's a disaccharide that's composed of glucose and fructose (see Figure 3).

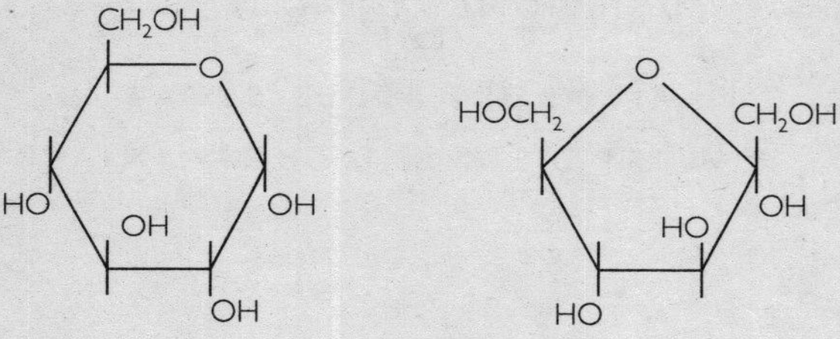

Glucose   Fructose

Figure 3: The chemical structures of glucose and fructose.

TYPES OF REFINED SUGAR

- White (granulated)
- Brown
- Confectioners (powdered)
- Raw
- Molasses
- Pancake syrup
- High fructose corn syrup
- Turbinado
- Maltodextrins

The natural sweetness of fruit and honey comes from mixtures of sugar, glucose and fructose. The mild sweetness of milk comes from another disaccharide, lactose, which is composed of glucose and galactose (Figure 4).

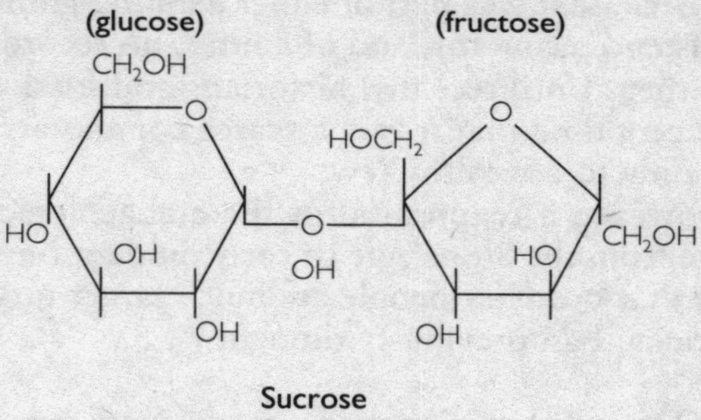

Sucrose

Figure 4: The chemical structure of sucrose (cane sugar).

Because sweetness comes from a mixture of sugars, not just sugar cane, we use many terms to define the original source:

- naturally-occurring sugars
- refined sugars
- added sugars
- concentrated sugars
- intrinsic and extrinsic sugars

If this confuses you, don't worry—it confuses the experts too!

HOW MUCH HONEY DID OUR ANCESTORS EAT?

It is possible that intakes of honey at various times during history may well have rivaled our current consumption of refined sugar.

In pre-industrial times, honey was the main source of concentrated sweetness in the diets of many people. There are no precise figures for honey consumption because it was part of either a hunter-gatherer or subsistence economy, and of course, no records were kept then. Until recently, historians and food writers have proposed that it was a scarce commodity available only to a wealthy few.

However, a reappraisal of the archaeological evidence from the Stone Age to early modern times suggests that ordinary people ate much larger quantities of honey than previously thought.

- The ancient Egyptians made frequent use of honey in their spiced breads, cakes and pastries, and for priming beer and wine.
- In Roman times, half of the recipes in a famous cookbook call for honey.
- In ancient Greece, those who died some distance from home were sometimes preserved in honey for transport.

All of this suggests that there was plenty of honey around. During medieval times we know that honey was sold in bulk quantities such as gallons and even barrels—units unlikely to be used for a scarce commodity. It was present in sufficient abundance to make mead, which was a common alcoholic drink made from honey.

Even the poorest people could have had access to honey because bees often made their hives in hollow logs or broken pots. Wealthy landowners might own dozens of beautifully constructed beehives and employ a beekeeper (Figure 5).

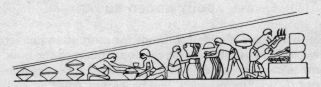

Figure 5: Ancient Egyptians made frequent use of honey.

Refined sugar may not have displaced more nutrient-rich items from our present-day diets but it may have displaced the only nutritionally comparable food—honey.

THE SUGAR-FAT SEESAW

Did you know that fat and sugar tend to show a reciprocal or seesaw relationship in the diet? Research shows that diets high in fat are low in sugar, and diets low in fat are high in sugar. But studies over the past decade have found that diets high in sugar are no less nutritious than low sugar diets. This is because restricting sugar is frequently followed by higher fat consumption, and most fatty foods are poor sources of nutrients.

In some cases, high sugar diets have been found to have higher micronutrient contents. This is because sugar is often used to sweeten some very nutritious foods, such as yogurts, breakfast cereals and milk.

A low sugar (and high fat) diet has more proven disadvantages than a high sugar (and low fat) diet.

■ ■ ■

ALL ABOUT ADDED SUGAR

Refined sugar is added to foods for more than just its sweetness. For example, sugar contributes to the bulk and texture of cakes and cookies and provides viscosity and "mouth feel" in beverages such as soft drinks and fruit juices. Sugar is also a powerful preservative and contributes to the long storage life of jams and confectionery.

In frozen products like ice cream, sugar has multiple functions: It acts as an emulsifier, preventing the separation of the water and fat phases; it lowers the freezing point, thereby making the product more liquid and "creamier" at the temperature at which it's eaten.

What's more, sugar retards the crystallization of the lactose in dairy foods and milk chocolate (tiny crystals of lactose feel like sand on the tongue).

In canned fruit, sugar syrups are used to prevent mushiness caused by the osmotic movement of sugar out of the fruit and into the surrounding fluid. Because sugar masks unpleasant flavors, sugar syrups are used as carriers for drugs and medicines, especially for young children who are unable to swallow tablet formulations.

In products such as yogurt and coffee, sugar masks the acidity or bitterness; it also balances the sugar-acid ratio in fruit juices and cordials.

Microorganisms also use sugar as the energy source for fermentation, so sugar is often deliberately added to foods for that purpose. It's added for the yeast in bread- and beer-making, but is totally converted to alcohol and other products in the process, so we don't end up consuming it as sugar.

■ ■ ■

WHAT ABOUT LOW CALORIE PRODUCTS?

It's difficult to produce low calorie products because refined sugar is added to foods for so many reasons—not just for sweetness. So when manufacturers design a low calorie, low sugar product they find that many substances (e.g., preservatives, emulsifiers, antioxidants) need to be added to perform all the roles that sugar did alone.

LOW FAT DIETS AND SUGAR INTAKE

One of the most important implications of the sugar-fat seesaw is that recommendations to reduce both sugar and fat may be counterproductive.

Most people are surprised to learn that the foods that provide most of our sugar intake (e.g. soft drinks, dairy products, breakfast cereals) are often low in fat. Similarly, the foods that provide most of our fat (e.g. meat, butter/margarine, fried foods) are often very low in sugar.

You may well be wondering how people in less affluent areas like Africa and China manage without sugar and still manage to eat a low fat diet. While it's true that they eat a low fat, low sugar diet, their actual diet is far from balanced and optimal—their total energy and micronutrient intake is lower than it should be, often resulting in compromised growth and nutrition. High starch diets are not a recipe for lifelong health and longevity.

Research shows that reducing your fat intake (especially that of saturated fat) is certainly more likely to result in desirable changes in body weight, blood lipids, insulin sensitivity and cardiovascular risk factors. But trying to reduce your sugar intake at the same time may not only compromise the effort to reduce fat, but reduce the palatability of your diet, and consequently the likelihood that you'll be able to stay on it over the long haul.

■

HIGH STARCH DIETS ARE NOT A RECIPE FOR LIFELONG HEALTH AND LONGEVITY.

■

Chapter 4

IS OUR LIKING FOR SWEETNESS INSTINCTUAL?

THE ROLE OF SUGAR IN OUR DIET

IS THERE SUCH A THING AS
A SUGAR CRAVING?

THE RISE OF REFINED SUGAR

HOW MUCH SUGAR DO WE EAT?

Sugars in fruit and honey have provided carbohydrate energy in human diets for millions of years—ever since primates began evolving on a steady diet of fruit and berries in the rainforests of Africa 50 million years ago.

Our appreciation for the "sweet" sensation runs deep in the human psyche. In literature and mythology, sweetness is linked with pleasure and goodness, and in everyday language we use terms associated with sweetness to describe the things we love (sweetie pie, honeymoon). Our first food, breast milk, is sweet—in fact the sweetest of all mammalian milks. Infants smile when you offer them a sweet solution and cry if you give them something sour or bitter.

Sweetness is not a learned taste: Everyone could be said to be born with a sweet tooth. Scientists don't know why we seem to prefer sweetness, but it may be related to our brain's dependence on glucose as its sole source of fuel. Perhaps those early human beings who were most able to detect sweetness were those most likely to survive. In fact, modern day monkeys that seek out fruit and berries have larger brains than those that survive on the leaves close at hand.

Our hunter-gatherer ancestors relished honey and other sources of concentrated sugars such as maple syrup, dried fruit and honey ants. Wild honey was so highly prized that they went to great lengths to obtain it.

SOME SOURCES OF SUGAR IN EARLY HUMAN DIETS

- Honey
- Parts of insects
- Honey ants
- Grape sugar
- Dates
- Maple syrup
- Sorghum
- Maize
- Sugar beets
- Sugar cane

As we mentioned earlier, our present use of refined sugars replaces our previous reliance on honey. In contrast, starches (the other form of carbohydrate energy) played a relatively minor role in human diets until we started cultivating staples such as wheat and corn some 10,000 years ago.

■

SUGARS IN FRUIT AND HONEY PROVIDED THE ONLY CARBOHYDRATE ENERGY IN HUMAN DIETS FOR MILLIONS OF YEARS.

■

SOURCES OF STARCH

- Breads
- Breakfast cereals
- Rice
- Potatoes, potato chips
- Snack foods
- Peas
- Legumes (dried peas and beans)
- Cakes
- Cookies

THE ROLE OF SUGAR IN OUR DIET

Sugar plays a unique role in our diet. No other nutrient satisfies our natural (instinctual) desire for sweetness. There are also some healthy reasons to include a reasonable amount of sugar in your diet. It will help you:

- maintain an ideal weight
- reduce your intake of saturated fat
- maximize your micronutrient intake

Sugar also serves other roles in our food supply, too. It acts as a preservative, adds texture and improves the flavors of many foods. When we take the sugar out of foods we have to add other ingredients to do the job: We sometimes need intense sweeteners that help to replace the original sweetness; fat or maltodextrins to replace the bulk and texture; or preservatives to replace sugar's anti-microbial properties.

WHAT IS A REASONABLE INTAKE?

A reasonable intake of sugar would come to no more than about 12½ to 15 teaspoons of refined sugar a day. (Since we already eat too much sugar, it would be a good idea for most of us to stick to the lower end of that range.) That amount includes all sources of refined sugar—in soft drinks, candy, cakes, cookies and frozen desserts, as well as what we add ourselves to tea, coffee and breakfast cereals.

IS THERE SUCH A THING AS A SUGAR CRAVING?

The notion that we can become addicted to sugar and crave it constantly is based on the false assumption that sugar causes wild fluctuations in blood sugar— that it sends blood sugar levels soaring, floods the system with sugar and creates rebound or reactive "hypoglycemia" (low blood sugar levels). The low blood sugar is claimed to be responsible for the "craving."

This simply isn't true. Many studies show that

most sugary foods cause very moderate rises in blood sugar. Some types of bread and potatoes produce higher blood sugar levels than sugar. But no one ever hears about potato addiction!

If we crave sugar, it's because we humans have an instinctual liking for it—part of the hard wiring in our brains tells us that sweet foods are a safe form of energy. If we deny this instinct by deliberately restricting sweet food, it's not surprising that we find ourselves wanting it.

Studies of people who claimed to crave sugar actually found that the preferred foods were sweet-fat combinations such as cakes and cookies, which contain more energy as fat than they do as sugar.

Women appear to like these sweet-fat combinations more than men, who prefer meat and starch-fat combinations such as baked potatoes. This female preference may be related to a woman's greater requirement for carbohydrate during pregnancy and lactation. The fetus uses only glucose as a source of fuel (fat can't cross the placenta) and is entirely dependent on the mother for this glucose. During lactation, women secrete up to 70 grams of carbohydrate a day in the form of the sugar in milk.

So, if you think you have a sugar craving, you don't have to beat it or bust it. Enjoy!

■

IF YOU HAVE A SUGAR CRAVING
YOU DON'T HAVE TO BEAT IT OR BUST IT.
ENJOY!

■

THE RISE OF REFINED SUGAR

Refined sugar is also known as table sugar, cane sugar or beet sugar. Sugar cane was one of the first foods that we began to cultivate deliberately (no prize for guessing why!). Sugar cane was first grown in Papua New Guinea 10,000 years ago, and the practice spread gradually to Egypt (2,300 years ago), Arabia (1,300 years ago) and Japan (1,100 years ago). Sugar beet, the main source of refined sugar in cool climates, was first cultivated in Europe 500 years ago.

Sugar cane and sugar beet have a naturally high content of sugar (about 16 percent) and have been commercially exploited as concentrated sources of sugar since 1600. Unfortunately, slaves harvested the crops, and were the main source of labor. Prior to this, refined sugar was a rare and expensive commodity and honey was much cheaper.

Sugar consumption increased dramatically in Europe beginning in the second half of the 18th century and replaced honey as the major source of sweetness. Our consumption levels peaked around 1900 and have remained, with minor variations, much the same for the past 100 years. Since 1970, though, corn syrup solids (glucose syrups made from hydrolyzed corn starch) and high-fructose corn syrup have partially replaced some of the refined sugar in manufactured products.

■

SOFT DRINKS (10 TO 12 PERCENT SUGAR) ARE LESS CONCENTRATED SOURCES OF SUGAR THAN EITHER SUGAR CANE OR SUGAR BEET (16 PERCENT SUGAR).

■

HOW MUCH SUGAR DO WE EAT?

According to the USDA's Human Nutrition Research Center, Americans eat an average of 20 teaspoons of added sugar a day—or about 16 percent of calories.

Unfortunately, this amount is higher than the amount considered acceptable by health authorities all over the world, including those in the United States. Public health experts suggest that our intake should be no more than 12½ to 15 teaspoons of added sugar a day, or about 10 to 12 percent of total calories. (It's a good idea for most of us to stick to the lower end of those ranges, since we already tend to eat too much sugar.)

Use the menus on pages 41 to 44 to help bring your sugar intake back in line with international guidelines.

Chapter 5

THE IMPORTANCE OF BLOOD SUGAR

THE FATE OF SUGAR IN YOUR BODY

BLOOD SUGAR RESPONSES AFTER A MEAL

A normal blood sugar (glucose) level is our life-line. It allows our brains, red cells and other systems to function properly. If our blood sugar levels drop too low, brain function is compromised and we suffer a range of symptoms, including sweating and nausea.

On the other hand, if blood sugar levels are too high for too long, then our eyesight, kidneys and heart function are affected. We get the glucose in our blood from our diets and from the liver, where it's synthesized.

■ ■ ■

BLOOD SUGAR OR BLOOD GLUCOSE?

Blood sugar and blood glucose mean exactly the same thing. In this book we use the term blood sugar because it is the one most familiar to the public.

Consuming sugar (and any other carbohydrate that includes starch) produces hormonal responses that not only help the body take up this new source of energy and but also limit the rise in blood sugar levels.

Insulin plays an important role in bringing blood sugar levels back to normal after a meal by "opening the gates" and transporting glucose from the blood into the cells. Insulin also signals the liver to stop making glucose molecules and halts the breakdown of fat as a source of energy.

During the 3 to 4 hours after a meal, the amount of carbohydrate we consume (whether as starch or sugar) far exceeds the amount of carbohydrate that our cells are able to oxidize. As a result, much of the dietary carbohydrate-derived glucose is stored as glycogen in the liver and skeletal muscles and is subsequently released and oxidized within the next 12 hours.

That means that what happens to sugar in your body is the same as with all other dietary carbohydrates. The carbohydrates:

- oxidize (burn) in the tissues as a source of energy
- are stored as glycogen in liver and muscle cells
- get recycled in the liver for the synthesis of new glucose molecules (this is quite an active pathway)

■ are converted and stored as fat mainly in the liver (under unusual circumstances only)

The body's glycogen reserves are small (usually one-half to one pound for a 110- to 154-pound adult; higher in trained athletes). The capacity to store more can be developed by exercise, training and diet.

A normal diet provides about 200 to 300 grams of carbohydrate a day. So within any 24-hour period, our bodies have totally oxidized the absorbed dietary carbohydrate, including sugar. Other body processes that help us dispose of dietary carbohydrate, such as conversion into fat or nonessential amino acids, are relatively unimportant in comparison.

THE FATE OF SUGAR IN YOUR BODY

The stomach empties the mix of foods and digestive enzymes into the small intestine where sugar is digested. The enzyme responsible for sugar digestion is called sucrase, which is located in the lining of the small intestine. The enzyme digests sucrose into glucose and fructose which are then absorbed into the bloodstream. Much of the sugar we add to foods has already been broken down prior to consumption; in fact, we actually swallow a mixture of glucose, fructose and sucrose. Soft drinks are a good example.

The glucose molecule derived from sugar digestion is transported rapidly into the bloodstream while fructose is absorbed much more slowly. So slowly, in fact, that a large quantity of fructose (more than one ounce) by itself will cause diarrhea. The high fructose content of apple juice has been blamed for "toddler diarrhea."

Once absorbed into the bloodstream, glucose and fructose travel to the liver where some of the glucose and virtually all the fructose is removed. The body then burns the fructose as an immediate source of energy, while glucose passes into the circulation, entering the muscles and other tissues under the influence of the hormone insulin. In the muscle cells, glucose displaces fat as the source of energy and is burned to carbon dioxide and water. Under normal circumstances very little of the glucose is converted to fat.

BLOOD SUGAR RESPONSES AFTER A MEAL

After a meal containing sugar or starch, the blood sugar rises and reaches a peak within 15 to 30 minutes, then returns to baseline within 2 hours. In people with diabetes, this peak occurs later—between 45 and 60 minutes after the meal because there is a relative deficiency of insulin. In the past, scientists assumed that refined sugar caused a more rapid rise in blood glucose levels than starchy foods or naturally occurring sources of sugars like fruit. Further research has proven this assumption *incorrect*.

Most starchy foods, including potatoes, bread and many breakfast cereals are digested and absorbed rapidly and the blood sugar response is almost as high as that seen with an equivalent amount of pure glucose. Foods containing refined sugar, such as soft drinks and ice cream, have been shown to give moderate rises in blood sugar, on average less than that of bread. (Remember, though: Americans in general need to eat less sugar. Let this book help you follow more reasonable guidelines.)

In addition, the blood sugar response to some foods containing refined sugars is similar to that of foods containing naturally occurring sugars (Figure 6).

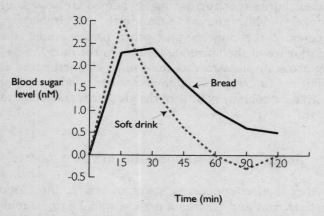

Figure 6: Comparison of blood sugar responses after 50 grams of carbohydrate in the form of sucrose or bread. (Notice the line for bread is higher from 15 to 120 minutes; this prolonged interval of increased blood sugar actually creates an *excess* of blood sugar over a extended period of time.)

Chapter 6

GLYCEMIC INDEX TABLES FOR SUGAR AND ENERGY

FOODS CONTAINING REFINED SUGAR

FOODS WITH NATURALLY OCCURRING SUGARS

STARCHY FOODS WITH LITTLE OR NO SUGAR

As we mentioned earlier, the glycemic index is used to classify foods according to their ability to raise the level of sugars in the blood, and we test all foods in equivalent carbohydrate portions according to standardized methodology. The following tables show the G.I. values of a range of common foods.

. . .

Foods Containing Refined Sugar	G.I.
Bakery Goods	
Angel food cake	67
Apple muffin	44
Blueberry muffin	59
Banana bread	47
Cookies	
Graham crackers	74
Milk Arrowroot	69
Oatmeal	55
Shortbread	64
Social Tea	55
Vanilla wafer	77
Breakfast Cereals	
All-Bran with extra fiber	51
Cheerios	74
Cocoa Krispies	77
Corn Flakes	84
Crispix	87
Muesli, toasted	43
Muesli, non-toasted	56
Raisin Bran	73
Rice Krispies	82
Dairy Foods	
Ice cream, 10% fat	61
Ice cream, low fat	50
Milk, chocolate, 1%	34
Pudding	43
Yogurt, nonfat, fruit flavored, with sugar	33
Candy	
Jelly beans	80

Foods Containing Refined Sugar	G.I.
Life Savers, peppermint	70
Mars Bar	65
Milk chocolate bar	49
Sports Drinks	
Gatorade	78
Isostar	73
Sportsplus	74
Soft Drinks	
Fanta	68
Coca Cola	63
Spreads	
Nutella	33
Jams	48–55

Foods Containing Naturally Occurring Sugars	G.I.
Apple	38
Apple juice	40
Apricots, fresh	57
Apricots, dried	31
Banana	55
Cantaloupe	65
Cherries	22
Dates, dried	103
Grapefruit	25
Grapefruit juice, unsweetened	48
Grapes, green	46
Kiwi	52
Mango	55
Orange	44

Foods Containing Naturally Occurring Sugars	G.I.
Orange juice	46
Peach	28
Pear	38
Pineapple	66
Pineapple juice, unsweetened	46
Plums	39
Raisins	64
Watermelon	72

Starchy Foods with Little or No Sugar	G.I.

Breads

Dark rye, Schinkenbrot	86
French baguette	95
Hamburger bun	61
Kaiser roll	73
Light rye	68
Natural Ovens 100% whole grain	51
Pita bread, whole wheat	57
Pumpernickel	51
Rye bread	65
Sourdough	52
Sourdough rye	57
Stoneground whole wheat	53
White	70

Cereal Grains

Barley, pearled	25
Buckwheat groats (kasha)	54
Bulgur, cooked	48
Couscous, cooked	65
Cornmeal, whole grain	68

STARCHY FOODS WITH LITTLE OR NO SUGAR	G.I.
Sweet corn, canned	55
Taco shells	68

Rice
Basmati, white	58
Brown	55
Converted, Uncle Ben's	44
Instant	87
Long grain, white	56
Short grain, white	72

Crackers
Kavli	71
Premium soda crackers	74
Rice cakes	82
Ryvita	69
Stoned wheat thins	67
Water cracker	78

Pasta
Capellini	45
Fettucine	32
Gnocchi	68
Linguine, thick	46
Linguine	55
Macaroni	45
Macaroni and cheese dinner	64
Ravioli, meat filled	39
Spaghetti, white	41
Spaghetti, whole wheat	37
Spirali durum	43
Star Pastina	38
Tortellini (cheese)	50
Vermicelli	35

Starchy Foods with Little or No Sugar	G.I.
Potatoes	
Desirée, boiled	101
French fries	75
Instant potato	86
New, boiled	62
New, canned	61
Red-skinned, microwaved	79
Sebago, boiled	87
White-skinned, baked	85
Legumes and Beans	
Soy beans, boiled	18
Lima beans baby, frozen	32
Lentils, green and brown, boiled	30
Lentils, red, boiled	26
Black beans, boiled	30
Butter beans, boiled	31
Chickpeas, canned, drained	42
Chickpeas, boiled	33
Navy beans, boiled	38
Split peas, yellow, boiled	32
Snacks	
Potato chips	54
Pretzels	83

Note: The full G.I. Table appears in Chapter 17.

LABEL READING 101

Not sure if a food you're buying is high in sugar? Check the ingredient list on the label. If you see several of these words, or if any is listed as a first or second ingredient, you're probably buying a high-sugar product.

- corn sweetener
- dextrose
- fructose
- fruit juice concentrate
- glucose
- honey
- lactose
- maltose
- molasses
- sugar

Chapter 7

EXPERT OPINIONS

WHAT THESE RECOMMENDATIONS MEAN

DON'T GO OVERBOARD

LOW G.I., REASONABLE SUGAR MENUS

*E*xperts from many countries have studied sugar's overall effect on health, including the United Nation's Food and Agriculture Organization (FAO) and the World Health Organization (WHO). A FAO/WHO group concluded that:

- Reasonable intake of sugar-rich foods can help to create a palatable and nutritious diet.

In addition, the American panel concluded that:

- At the levels normally consumed, sugar has no effect on disease risk, apart from dental cavities.

WHAT THESE RECOMMENDATIONS MEAN

That means you should consume no more than about 12½ to 15 teaspoons of sugar per day from sources including soft drinks, breakfast cereals and bakery products. As we discussed earlier, the average level of consumption in the U.S. is slightly above this target, so stick closer to 12½ teaspoons or less, if possible.

The difficulty is that the public and some health authorities, however, remain concerned about the health effect of sugars especially in relation to diabetes and dental disease.

DON'T GO OVERBOARD!

We don't mean to suggest that you should indulge in an excessive amount of sugar simply because sugar restriction is unnecessary. Far from it! But we do want to take the pressure off. Your normal instincts should guide you to eat a reasonable quantity of sugar—about 10 to 12 percent of calories a day.

To give you a guide to what this means in practice we have provided the following menu and a list of the refined sugar contents of a range of common foods.

A ONE-DAY MENU CONTAINING A REASONABLE QUANTITY OF SUGAR

Breakfast
    1½ cups All Bran with extra fiber and 1 teaspoon sugar
    2 slices 100% stoneground whole wheat toast with margarine
    Coffee with 1% milk and 1 teaspoon of sugar

Snack
   3 Social Tea biscuits
   Tea

Lunch
   Ham and reduced fat cheddar cheese sandwich on
      grain bread
   An apple
   8 ounces unsweetened orange juice

Snack
   A pear
   Water

Dinner
   Steak with potato, peas, carrots and corn
   2 scoops low fat ice cream
   Water or unsweetened tea

Snack
   No sugar added hot chocolate with ½ cup mini-
   marshmallows

This menu contains about 50 grams (about 12½ teaspoons) of added sugar.

   The menu on pages 41 to 42 provides 1900 calories and meets the recommended proportions of
nutrients, with 24 percent energy coming from fat
(recommendation: less than 30 percent) and 57 percent of energy coming from carbohydrate (recommendation: more than 50 percent).
   The total carbohydrate content is 285 grams made
up of 123 grams starch plus 155 grams sugars (60
grams added, 95 grams naturally occurring).

A REASONABLE QUANTITY OF SUGAR
IN A 10-YEAR-OLD CHILD'S DIET

Breakfast
1 cup of Coco Pops with 1% milk
½ banana
4 ounces unsweetened fruit juice

Lunch
2 slices rye bread with 1 ounce ham with mustard,
   lettuce and tomato
1 small apple
Water

Snack
1 cup of homemade popcorn
1 cup of reduced fat milk

Dinner
½ cup spaghetti with meat sauce
Carrot and celery sticks
½ cup vanilla pudding with ½ unsweetened sliced
   peach
Water

This child's menu provides about 40 grams (10 teaspoons) of refined sugars. It provides 1500 calories
with 25 percent of energy from fat and 58 percent of
energy from carbohydrate.

■ ■ ■

A LOW G.I. MENU FOR SOMEONE
WITH DIABETES CONTAINING
A REASONABLE QUANTITY OF SUGAR

Breakfast
    1 cup of rolled oats with 1% milk and 1 teaspoon
      of brown sugar
    A fresh orange
    Tea or coffee with 1% milk

Snack
    2 gingersnaps
    Tea or coffee with 1% milk

Lunch
    A mixed grain sandwich filled with 2 tablespoons
      natural peanut butter
    8 ounces nonfat fruit yogurt
    Water

Dinner
    Pan-fried fish with spinach, tomato and onion
      served over a cup of long-grain white rice
    Green salad
    Tea or coffee with 1% milk

Snack
    ½ cup low fat ice cream with unsweetened canned
      pears

This menu contains 40 grams (10 teaspoons) of added sugar. The total energy content is 1550 calories; 22 percent of energy is from fat, 55 percent from carbohydrate. The fat content is 38 grams. The total carbohydrate content is 220 grams, with 112 grams from starch and 108 grams from sugars (added plus naturally occurring).

REFINED SUGAR CONTENT OF VARIOUS FOODS (GRAMS)

1 rounded teaspoon of sugar	6
1 tablespoon of jam	8
1 tablespoon of honey	20
5 squares chocolate	20
1 chocolate bar (average)	35
12 ounce can of soft drink (average)	45
1 cup of sweetened fruit juice	5
1 ounce undiluted cordial	18
1 granola bar (average)	8
2 Lorna Doone shortbread cookies	3
1 cream filled sandwich cookie	5
1 piece of chocolate cake	11
1 cinnamon and sugar doughnut	7
1 piece of plain cake	7

Sources of refined sugars

Soft drinks, cordials and fruit juice drinks

Sweetened dairy products (ice cream, yogurt, flavored milk, pudding)

Milk flavorings (such as Nestle's Quik)

Sweetened breakfast cereals

Flavored toppings

Jams, honey, pancake syrup, Nutella

Cakes, cookies and bakery products

Candy and chocolate

Frozen desserts (such as Popsicles, Fudgesicles and Italian ices)

Table sugars: white, raw, brown, cube

Sources of naturally occurring sugars

Sugar cane
Fruit of any sort
Honey
Dried fruit (dates, raisins)
Breast milk (lactose)
Cow's milk (lactose)
Vegetables (some are higher than others, such as carrots, red peppers, tomatoes, sweet corn and beets)
Maple syrup

Chapter 8

DOES SUGAR PROMOTE ILLNESS?

CANDIDA AND THRUSH (YEAST) INFECTIONS

DIABETES

BLOOD CHOLESTEROL

BEHAVIOR CHANGES

MEMORY

CANCER

SUGAR AND NUTRITIONAL DEFICIENCIES

O ld myths die hard: Sugar has been implicated in either the promotion or exacerbation of any number of illnesses for years. But according to the United Nations FAO/WHO Expert Consultation on Carbohydrates (1998), "there is no evidence of a direct involvement of sucrose, other sugars and starch in the etiology of lifestyle-related diseases." Still, the fiction persists. Below, we discuss a few conditions for which some people think sugar is to blame, and the science that finally clears sugar's name for good.

■ ■ ■

CANDIDA AND THRUSH (YEAST) INFECTIONS

Many natural health therapists claim that high-sugar diets promote the growth of yeast infections of the vagina, mouth and skin. While infections caused by Candida albicans are very common, there is absolutely no evidence that a diet high in sugars causes the infection or influences it in any way.

The Candida organism is in our bodies all the time. The infection comes from its uncontrolled growth. Antibiotics are often the culprit, because they inhibit the bacteria that normally control yeast numbers. You know you have too much yeast if you experience itching and burning sensations.

One of the reasons sugar is often heard in connection with Candida is that people with diabetes are particularly prone to infection with this organism. When blood sugars are abnormally high, as in uncontrolled diabetes, the sugars spill over into the urine and create a good place for the organism to grow. But because starches increase blood sugars to the same (or greater) extent than sugary foods, potatoes and bread would have to be incriminated in Candida infections too!

■

RESEARCH HAS SHOWN THAT CERTAIN BLOOD MARKERS OF DIABETES CONTROL WERE DIRECTLY RELATED TO THE DIET'S GLYCEMIC INDEX: THOSE PEOPLE WITH HIGHER SUGAR INTAKE HAD THE BEST DIABETES CONTROL.

■

DIABETES

Diabetes associations worldwide have now recognized that there is no need to strictly avoid refined sugar. This change of heart resulted from the unarguable scientific evidence that blood sugar responses after eating sugary foods were no higher than that of starchy staples such as bread.

In longer term studies in people with diabetes, those who were required to eat 12½ teaspoons of refined sugar a day in tea and coffee had no higher average blood sugars than those people given artificial sweeteners. Even extremely large amounts of sugar (75 teaspoons) didn't compromise blood sugar control. We definitely don't recommend this amount: It just proves a point.

There's no evidence to suggest that refined sugar causes worsening of glucose tolerance, insulin sensitivity or diabetes risk in humans. There are studies in rats that support this idea, but the amounts of sugar fed to the rats (equivalent to 100 or more cans of soft drink a day) are so much higher than a human would ever eat or want to eat, that the findings are really irrelevant. When rats are fed sugar at the upper levels of human consumption, scientists have noted no adverse effects.

The important point is that avoiding sugar has consequences of its own that can be far more serious than any potential effects of eating refined sugar. In other words, restricting sugar may actually be counterproductive in people with diabetes. This is because of the sugar-fat seesaw (restricting sugar is frequently followed by higher fat consumption) and because starchy foods often have a high glycemic index.

Past studies in people with diabetes have clearly shown that they eat less sugar but more saturated fat than the general population. The consequence, of course, is that they die of heart disease caused by hardening of the arteries. Some of you may be thinking that we should all try harder to restrict both sugar and fat, but this means people should eat more starchy foods to fill the gap.

The trouble is, some starchy foods have a more beneficial effect on blood sugars than others. If starchy foods with a high glycemic index (such as some types of bread and potatoes) fill the hole left by sugar, then it may do more harm than good. Unlike sugar, high G.I. starchy foods have been associated with increased risk of diabetes and heart disease in the general population.

Two large studies from Harvard School of Public Health involving 65,000 female nurses and 50,000 male health professionals, showed that high G.I., low fiber diets were associated with double the risk of type 2 diabetes. What's more, in the Nurses' Study, heart attack risk was doubled in those people who ate a high G.I. diet. The harmful consequences for people with diabetes are likely to be greater still.

THE OFFICIAL POSITION

In 1994, the American Diabetes Association published a position statement declaring that the use of sucrose in a diabetes meal plan does not impair blood glucose control. They said that calories from sugar must be included as part of a diabetic's overall carbohydrate intake.

■

UNLIKE SUGAR, HIGH G.I. STARCHY FOODS HAVE BEEN
ASSOCIATED WITH INCREASING THE RISK OF DIABETES
AND HEART DISEASE IN THE GENERAL POPULATION.

■

BLOOD CHOLESTEROL

Most readers will be aware that high blood cholesterol levels increase our risk of a heart attack. The
dietary component most clearly associated with
increasing cholesterol levels is saturated fat; reducing
saturated fat is the most effective way to reduce the
risk of heart attack.

Sugar, on the other hand, has never been found to
increase cholesterol levels. When we reduce saturated
fat, we tend to eat more carbohydrate to replace the
missing calories. In some studies, this increase in carbohydrate intake—either from starches or sugars—
has been found to cause a rise in blood triglyceride
levels and a fall in the "good" form of cholesterol, or
HDL. That's not good, since these factors can act
independently of cholesterol levels to increase our
risk of heart disease.

High levels of "bad" blood fats, such as triglycerides, and low levels of HDL are especially harmful
for people with diabetes, who more often than not
have a high risk of heart disease despite normal blood
cholesterol levels. As a result, some experts suggest
that the best course of action is to avoid both saturated fat and large amounts of carbohydrate and to
eat monounsaturated fat instead.

The push for eating more monounsaturated fat is why experts and the media promote diets high in olive oil. Indeed, people in Mediterranean countries who do eat more unsaturated fat and less carbohydrate than other industrialized countries have a low risk of heart disease. But their diet and lifestyle differ in many other ways that may act in unison to reduce heart disease risk.

For example, people in Mediterranean countries eat more fruit and vegetables, more pasta and legumes, more salads and vinaigrette dressings. All of these foods have a low glycemic index, so blood sugar levels are low. Also, because of these low G.I. foods, there's less of a tendency for the carbohydrate to increase triglycerides and reduce HDL levels. That said, it becomes more clear that olive oil alone is not responsible for the reduced risk of heart disease in Mediterranean countries.

Some nutrition experts are concerned that diets high in sugar might increase triglycerides more than other carbohydrates can. The basis of this worry? Studies that incorporate very large amounts of sugars (providing one-third or more of total calories) have found higher triglycerides and lower HDL than when starch was eaten.

Furthermore, some people appear to be more sensitive to the effects of dietary sugars on blood fats than others. We need to examine these variations more closely before we can be absolutely clear about the role of sugar. In the meantime, however, you can be reassured that diets that contain more typical amounts of sugar (around 12 teaspoons—50 grams—a day or 10 percent of calories), have no special effect on blood fats.

■　■　■

■

WHEN WE REDUCE SATURATED FAT,
WE TEND TO EAT MORE CARBOHYDRATE
TO REPLACE THE MISSING CALORIES.

■

BEHAVIOR CHANGES

Some people believe that sugar causes ADD (attention deficit disorder, previously known as hyperactivity). That opinion is based on two theories:

- a possible allergic response to sugar, or
- a low blood sugar "rebound" after sugar consumption

However, results from many published research papers that have studied hundreds of people do not provide any support whatsoever for the idea that refined sugar causes or exacerbates ADD or affects cognitive performance in children. It's interesting to note that even those children originally considered to be adversely affected by sugar showed no effects when the sugar was given to them in a double-blind situation. (In this case, "double-blind" means that no one—including the scientist, the child and the parent—knew whether the child was getting sugar or an inactive substitute.)

It's possible that a very small number of children may have distinct reactions and respond adversely to sugar. But any carbohydrate, including bread and potatoes, could also be to blame if it causes blood sugar fluctuations.

Not only does sugar have no effect on most children's behavior, there's even some evidence that sugar might actually have a calming effect, if it has any effect at all: Glucose or sugar seems to influence the distress associated with painful procedures in human infants. In one study, babies given a heel prick cried less and had lower heart rates when they were given a 50 percent sugar solution just before the procedure than babies given plain water.

■

THERE IS SOME EVIDENCE THAT SUGAR MAY HAVE A CALMING EFFECT, IF IT HAS ANY EFFECT AT ALL.

■

MEMORY CHANGES

There is growing evidence that consuming glucose enhances learning and memory in both rats and humans. The effect is best demonstrated in elderly people and those with Alzheimer's, but is also seen in young adults, if the test is sufficiently difficult.

In one study, elderly people were asked to drink either a glucose- or saccharin-sweetened lemon drink and were then given a battery of neuropsychological tests that measured memory, overall intelligence, attention and motor functions. The glucose drink improved these folks' performance on both the logical and verbal memory part of the tests (there was no effect on attention).

In another study of university students, consuming glucose improved their recall of narrative prose by 40 percent.

CANCER

In the United Kingdom, an expert group recently released a major report about the nutritional aspects of the development of cancer. This report hardly mentions sugar at all. In the 15 pages of conclusions and recommendations, only two sentences include the word sugars as one of a group of "other nutrients" along with starch, folate, selenium, calcium, iron and zinc that might be involved in the causation or prevention of some cancers. The working party comments that there is not enough evidence to reach conclusions—either positive or negative—for any of these substances.

The committee recommended a balanced diet rich in cereals, fruits and vegetables. Sugar, when consumed within these dietary guidelines, is not implicated in cancer causation.

SUGAR AND NUTRITIONAL DEFICIENCIES

Many people think that eating refined and other added sugars is a bad idea because they offer "empty calories"—that is, they provide energy but without vitamins and minerals.

It's logical to assume that sugar dilutes the vitamin and mineral content of the diet but the real question is whether it happens in practice. If that were true, then we would expect to find that diets containing the least sugar would have the greatest quantities of micronutrients. But many large well-designed scientific studies found that diets containing moderately large amounts of added sugars were the most nutritious: more so than diets either low or very high in sugar. Researchers found that the higher the sugar content of the diet, the higher the intake of some micronutrients, including vitamins C, B_2 and calcium.

One of the reasons for this paradox is that sweetened foods can be excellent sources of micronutrients—breakfast cereals and dairy products such as flavored milk, yogurts and ice cream are good examples. People are more likely to eat them frequently and in larger quantities when they're sweetened. Many of us know children who refuse to drink plain milk but gobble down a strawberry milkshake or hot chocolate. A couple of teaspoons of brown sugar on oatmeal or a tablespoon of jam on toast encourages a child to eat nutritious, but otherwise fairly bland, foods.

The second reason that reasonable sugar intake equates with greater intake of micronutrients is the sugar-fat seesaw: That is, low sugar diets in practice are usually higher in fat. Fats such as cooking oils, butter and margarines are essentially empty calories, too. Of course, they do contain some vitamins, particularly the fat-soluble vitamins, but their very high calorie content means they tend to dilute rather than enrich the rest of the diet.

That isn't to say, of course, that *all* higher-sugar diets supply an adequate number of micronutrients. The fact is, most Americans eat too much added sugar already and too few servings of fruits and vegetables each day. So, though sugar is not a demon, we would do well to aim for at least five servings a day of fruits and vegetables and try to cut down on the amount of sugar we add to our food.

■

ADDED FATS, ALCOHOL, MODIFIED STARCHES AND EVEN PURE PROTEINS ARE OFTEN SOURCES OF "EMPTY CALORIES."

■

Chapter 9

SUGAR AND OBESITY

HOW WE STORE FAT
FEELINGS OF FULLNESS
THE FINAL TEST

There is a widespread belief that sugar is particularly associated with weight gain and obesity. This view stems largely from early studies in rats and mice that showed water sweetened with sugar led to rapid weight gain—not really surprising because water laced with any form of energy, whether it's amino acids, starch or fat would do the same thing, because all forms of food contain calories. Milk causes rapid weight gain, too! But the deed was done, and sugar's reputation for causing exceptional weight gain was accepted by the public and scientific community at large.

It's become clear that rats and humans are very different in respect to fat-making enzymes. Rodents are very efficient in converting carbohydrates (such as sugar or starch) into body fat, while humans have only limited quantities of the necessary enzymes and do it only under unusual circumstances.

HOW WE STORE FAT

We create human fat stores by channeling excess fat energy to fat storage, not by converting excess carbohydrate into fat. We know this because our fat stores have the very same fatty acid composition as our diet. If our diet is high in monounsaturated fat, then our fat stores will reflect this.

If we eat an excessive amount of carbohydrate energy, some of it will be stored as glycogen in our liver and muscles and all of it will eventually be burned (oxidized) as a fuel source.

If we overeat a very high carbohydrate diet (which is rather hard to do because it's often bulky and very filling), then it's the small amount of *fat* in the diet that will be channeled to fat storage.

Even an exceedingly large meal of pure glucose (500 grams, the equivalent of more than a gallon of soft drink in one hit) doesn't induce a net gain in fat. If overfeeding of glucose extends for several days, glycogen stores do become full (at about 1000 grams) and only at this point does sugar convert to fat. But this artificial situation is unlikely to occur outside the laboratory.

In everyday life, a high sugar intake causes an increase in feelings of fullness, so food intake is decreased.

■ ■ ■

FEELINGS OF FULLNESS

One of the most robust findings in recent nutrition science is that sugars result in much greater feelings of fullness compared to high-fat meals that contain the same number of calories.

In one study, students ate as much as they liked from a tasty smorgasbord of either high-sugar foods or high-fat foods on two separate occasions. They were "blind" to the nutrient content of the foods and the true purpose of the study. The investigators found that the students ate far fewer calories overall when they ate from the smorgasbord of high sugar foods.

In another study, students were given either a high-sugar or a high-fat snack and one hour later were allowed to eat from an array of appetizing foods. They ate significantly less when the earlier snack was high in sugars.

Scientists now say that fat is very easy to "passively overconsume." Of course a high-fat meal can make you feel full, even sickeningly so. But the point is, you would have to eat an excessively large number of calories before you'd feel full. We all know that it's all too easy to keep munching on those "addictive" high-fat foods such as chips and peanuts.

But we tend not to do the same thing with high sugar foods—eating jelly beans and other sugar confectionery is much more self-limiting—many of us feel a little nauseous if we indulge to excess.

THE FINAL TEST

The final test of the theory that "sugar makes you fat" is to look at the association between sugar intake and body weight in the general population. It's important that we exclude the dieters from such studies because they will tend to muddle the interpretation of the findings, having altered their diet in an effort to lose weight.

A well-designed study involving over 10,000 Scottish adults showed that diets low in sugars were associated with higher body mass index (a measure of overweight). In contrast, the diets high in sugars were associated with lower body weight. In fact, there was a consistent stepwise relationship between the two factors—the higher the sugar intake (as a percentage of calories or in grams per day), the lower the body mass index. This applied to both refined sugar and total sugars from all sources. This did not apply to starch—there was no difference in starch intake in lean and overweight people.

In a recent Australian study of identical twins, scientists found little evidence to associate any dietary factor with the degree of overweight. But, when the twins differed in weight by more than 9 pounds, the lighter twin tended to have a diet higher in sugar than the heavier twin.

We can cite many other studies that show this inverse association between sugars and weight status. Of course, all of them are open to the criticism that conscious or unconscious "under-reporting" of sugar by the heaviest people is responsible for the trend. However, the same can be said of fat under-reporting and yet fat shows a direct relationship to body weight in the same studies.

There's ample reason to incriminate high fat diets with overweight (passive overconsumption being one!), but no good scientific evidence to point the finger at sugar.

Chapter 10

SUGAR AND DENTAL HEALTH

MECHANISMS OF TOOTH DECAY

A WORD ABOUT LOW CALORIE SOFT DRINKS

*M*uch of what we know about the relationship of sugars to dental decay was gathered before the "fluoride era." Sugar's bad reputation seemed confirmed at that time when research showed a strong relationship between the number of decayed and missing teeth and the amount of sugar people ate.

In the post-fluoride era, it's clear that the best way to promote healthy teeth is to drink fluoridated water, floss daily, brush your teeth twice a day and use a fluoride toothpaste. Total sugar consumption has less to do with it than we once thought. Nowadays dentists recognize that all fermentable carbohydrates (i.e., both sugars and starches), can promote dental decay. More important, it's not the total amount eaten, but the frequency of eating and consistency of the food that determine its cavity-causing potential.

All fermentable carbohydrates, including sugars and starches, are capable of causing dental cavities. Naturally occurring sugars in breast milk, fruit and honey are no different from those in candies and other sweets, and whole grain cereals and flours are just as responsible. The starches in breakfast cereals and potatoes, when caught between the teeth, help to start dental cavities. That's why it makes no sense to suggest that we reduce our intake of sugar while simultaneously recommending higher starch intake.

Indeed, the first archaeological evidence of dental decay appeared 10,000 years ago when humans first adopted farming and starch became a common component of the diet (and long before refined sugar came along). Even in those days some people lost all of their teeth to dental decay.

MECHANISMS OF TOOTH DECAY

Every time we eat or drink, we subject our teeth to an unavoidable "acid wash" because the bacteria in plaque ferment any leftover carbohydrate that remains on teeth to acid.

Acid formation begins within minutes of eating and gradually dissolves the enamel of the tooth's surface, but teeth strengthened by fluoride have the best defense against this acid. For the following half hour after eating, the acids are gradually neutralized by saliva and the tooth surface returns to normal.

Dental experts have shown that our teeth can put up with about six of these "acid washes" a day and still stay in good shape. If you eat all your fermentable carbohydrates at breakfast, lunch, dinner, supper and snacks throughout the day, then your teeth should theoretically stay cavity-free.

However, sticky foods such as lollipops that remain on the teeth or stuck between them for long periods promote tooth decay because the acids are continually being formed by bacterial fermentation. Hard candies aren't the only culprit however—dried fruit and carbohydrates can stick between teeth too! (Foods like cornflakes can produce just as much acid as sugary foods.) Similarly, if we sip sweet drinks for hours (whether a soft drink or juice), we prolong the acid bath and increase the risk of cavities.

Some babies develop severe tooth decay by being continuously breastfed or bottle-fed throughout the night. If we eat very frequently, whether we're munching on non-sugary foods such as potato chips or naturally-occurring sugary foods such as fruit, we promote acid formation and dental decay. (In one study, dental decay was found to be significantly greater in citrus and other fruit pickers compared to the neighboring workers on vegetable farms!)

■

REGULAR TOOTH BRUSHING AND FLOSSING PLAY A MORE IMPORTANT ROLE IN THE PREVENTION OF TOOTH DECAY IN THE POST-FLUORIDE ERA.

■

Candies promote dental decay because you're more likely to eat them between meals than any other type of food. Furthermore, many types of confectionery take a long time to dissolve in the mouth (hard candies), are sticky (such as jelly beans and licorice) or are sucked for long periods (lollipops). There's no doubt that frequent consumption of these foods will promote tooth decay even in fluoridated areas. The actual amount of sugar eaten may be quite small, but the effect is enormous.

If we decide to replace these between-meal snacks with more "natural" products such as dried fruit, or with starchy foods such as bread and crackers, we may be no better off: It all comes down to frequency of consumption between meals.

Public health strategies to reduce the incidence of dental cavities are far more likely to be successful if they emphasize using fluoride toothpaste and practicing good dental hygiene, rather than reducing our sugar consumption.

A WORD ABOUT LOW CALORIE SOFT DRINKS

One of the most frequent ways people try to reduce their sugar intake is by drinking low calorie soft drinks in place of regular varieties. If, by doing this, the intention is to reduce dental cavities, this isn't the way to do it. Low calorie soft drinks are highly acidic, just like regular soft drinks and most fruits. The drink's acidic nature helps to dissolve the enamel on the tooth surface, even in the absence of bacteria and plaque. We've all heard the story of one famous brand of soft drink that completely dissolved a tooth overnight. Well, the same will happen with the regular or diet version of any soft drink.

The present trend to carry and drink water (both free and expensive versions) instead of juice or a soft drink is a good idea: Many people, much of the time, walk around in a state of semi-dehydration that affects both mental and physical performance!

Chapter 11

GOOD INTENTIONS

THE RISE OF SUGAR SUBSTITUTES
RID YOURSELF OF GUILT

One of the main messages of this book is that well-meaning efforts to reduce our sugar intake may do more harm than good. Unfortunately, when we reduce our consumption of sugar—either consciously or unconsciously—we tend to increase our intake of high G.I. foods (such as some types of bread and rice), or of foods high in saturated fat, such as cheese, crackers and potato chips. Those foods may do more long-term harm to our health than sugar ever will

While many nutritionists feel that people ought to be able to reduce both their sugar and fat intake to low levels, only a small minority of the population actually does so in practice. Furthermore, this recommendation is based on the assumed superiority of starches to sugars—that high intake of starchy foods such as some types of cereals, bread and potatoes always goes hand-in-hand with good health. Unfortunately, this isn't necessarily so—populations all over the world that have high starch intakes are among those with the highest rates of protein-energy malnutrition and stunted growth. Furthermore, starchy foods with high G.I. values increase insulin demand and therefore promote the diseases of affluence—diabetes, heart disease and obesity. Sugary foods have lower G.I. values than most starchy foods.

■

YOU CAN USE SUGAR TO MAXIMIZE YOUR WELL-BEING AND ENJOYMENT OF LIFE.

■

THE RISE OF SUGAR SUBSTITUTES

Our emphasis on reducing sugar intake also fuels the demand for intense sweeteners to use as sugar substitutes. In China, the relatively new soft drink industry is based almost entirely on saccharin-sweetened drinks not only because sugar is more expensive in China but also because it is seen as something that should be avoided. While there's no evidence that intense sweeteners cause harm, there is actually little support for using them at all. We're still an overweight nation despite the number of low calorie products that are on the market.

We spend millions of dollars on the research and development, safety testing and product development of foods incorporating intense sweeteners. In our opinion, this money would be better channeled into research on the real causes of obesity and diabetes and their treatment.

There may be a place for tooth-friendly candies made with sugar substitutes such as Isomalt, an artificial sweetener that's becoming more popular in the United States. Truth is, intense sweeteners are probably here to stay simply because nutrition and other health authorities continue to push the message that sugar is to be avoided if at all possible.

Our take-home message: Reasonable amounts of sugar (about 10 to 12 percent of total calories a day) need not be discouraged. That intake is associated with:

- the highest intake of micronutrients
- lower intakes of saturated fat
- a lower-G.I. diet
- a lower body weight

■

YOU DON'T NEED TO BEAT IT OR BUST IT,
AND YOU CAN CUT THE GUILT TRIP.
THE DESIRE FOR SWEETNESS IN FOODS
IS A HUMAN ONE.

■

RID YOURSELF OF GUILT

It's okay to use sugar if it improves the taste of those very nutritious but rather bland foods—low fat milk, yogurt, oatmeal and other whole grain breakfast cereals. Don't hesitate to put a tablespoon of jam on your bread, a little honey in your tea, or a sprinkle of sugar on unripe, sour or acidic fruit. And don't fret about the sugar in baked beans or canned fruit—these foods are good for you and if you are more likely to eat them because you like them sweetened, go ahead and enjoy.

It's a good nutritional rule of thumb to consider the nutrients your body will get from the nutrients you consume. Just don't forget your five servings of fruit and vegetables. If ice cream is your weak spot, choose low fat, not low sugar versions. If you want to "pig out" now and again—it's much better to do it on jelly beans and hard candies rather than on chocolate and potato chips.

Chaptewr 12

SECRETS TO LOW G.I. SNACKING

---

5 SNACKING TIPS

17 SUSTAINING SNACKS

*N*ow that you've had a chance to read about sugar and low G.I. foods, it's time to focus on snacking for a bit. Fact is, it's normal to get hungry and want to snack between your usual "three squares." Luckily, when you eat the low G.I. way there's no prohibition on between-meal nibbles. It's a great way to eat the foods you love without gaining weight!

Just remember that when you choose a between-meal bite, pick a low fat snack with a low glycemic index. For example, an apple with a glycemic index of 38 is better than a slice of white bread with a glycemic index of around 70, and will result in a smaller blood sugar jump.

New evidence suggests that the people who graze, eating small amounts of food throughout the day at frequent intervals, may actually be doing themselves a favor. Spreading the food out over longer periods of time will flatten out the peaks and valleys of blood glucose levels. So, snacking may be a good idea—as long as you don't overeat and gain weight.

Some snack foods with low G.I. values (such as peanuts, at 14) have a very high fat content and are not recommended for people trying to lose weight. As an occasional snack they are fine, especially because their fat is the healthier monounsaturated type. Just don't indulge in them every day. Remember, with peanuts, it's often hard to stop at just a handful!

5 SNACKING TIPS

- It is important to include a couple of servings of dairy foods each day for your calcium needs. If you haven't used yogurt or cheese in any meals, you may choose to make a low fat milkshake. One or two scoops of low fat ice cream or pudding can also boost your daily calcium intake.
- If you like whole grain breads, an extra slice makes a very good choice for a snack. Other snacks can include toasted sourdough English muffin halves, a waffle or a slice of raisin bread with a little butter.
- Fruit is always a low calorie option for snacks. You should try to consume at least 3 servings a day. It may be helpful to prepare fruit in advance to make it accessible and easy to eat.
- Ryvita whole grain crispbreads are a low calorie

snack if you want something dry and crunchy.
Popcorn (prepared at home using a minimum of
fat) is another good alternative.

- Keep vegetables (such as celery and carrot
  sticks, baby tomatoes, florets of blanched cauli-
  flower or broccoli) ready prepared.

SNACKING SUCCESS!

A recent study that compared people eating a diet of three
meals a day with those who had three meals and three snacks
showed that snacking stimulated the body to use up more
energy for metabolism compared with concentrating the same
amount of food into three meals. It's as if the more fuel you
give your body the more it will burn. Frequent small meals stim-
ulate the metabolic rate.

---

17 SUSTAINING SNACKS

- An apple
- An apple and oat bran muffin
- Dried apricots
- A mini can of baked beans
- A small bowl of cherries
- Ice cream (low fat) in a cone
- Milk, milkshake or smoothie (low fat, of course)
- Two or three oatmeal cookies
- An orange
- Six ounces of orange juice, freshly squeezed
- Pita bread spread with apple butter
- A big bowl of low fat popcorn

- One or 2 slices of raisin toast
- Whole grain bread sandwich with your favorite filling
- A bowl of Raisin Bran with skim milk
- A small box of raisins
- Six to 8 ounces of light yogurt

Chapter 13

THE LOW G.I. PANTRY

BREADS

BREAKFAST CEREALS

RICE AND GRAINS

LEGUMES

VEGETABLES

FRUITS

DAIRY FOODS

USEFUL FLAVORINGS, SAUCES AND
DRESSINGS

WHAT TO KEEP IN THE REFRIGERATOR AND
FREEZER

To make low G.I. choices easier, you need to keep the right foods in your cupboard. Here's a starter list for you to follow.

BREADS

If you're the only one in the house who will eat the "birdseed bread," keep a loaf in the freezer and pull out slices as you need them.

- 100% stoneground whole wheat
- Arnold's rye
- Banana bread
- Chapati (baisen)

- Natural Ovens 100% Whole Grain**
- Natural Ovens Happiness**
- Natural Ovens Hunger Filler**
- Natural Ovens Natural Wheat**
- Sourdough
- Sourdough rye
- Whole grain pumpernickel
- Whole wheat pita

**Natural Ovens breads are available in the United States through mail order. See the "For More Information" section for ordering information.

BREAKFAST CEREALS

- Kellogg's All-Bran with extra fiber
- Kellogg's Bran Buds with Psyllium
- Muesli (low fat varieties, read the labels)
- Rolled or old-fashioned oats
- Oat bran
- Rice bran
- Oatmeal

RICE AND GRAINS

- Pearled barley
- Basmati rice, brown or long-grain rice
- Uncle Ben's Converted rice
- Pasta of various shapes and flavors
- Noodles

LEGUMES

- Cooked lentils (red or brown), chickpeas, split peas
- Dried lentils, chickpeas, cannellini beans
- A variety of canned legumes (kidney beans, mixed beans, baked beans, lentils, chickpeas, black beans, pinto beans, butter beans, broad beans, chana dal)

VEGETABLES

All vegetables are good for you—fresh, frozen, and canned. Raw salad vegetables are available partially prepared to make a quick addition to the meal. Here are some low G.I. veggie varieties:

- Peas
- Sweet corn
- Sweet potato
- Canned new potatoes
- Carrots

Other canned vegetables such as tomatoes, asparagus, peas, mushrooms are handy to boost the vegetable content of a meal. Other convenient products are:

- Tomato paste
- Tomato purée
- Bottled tomato pasta sauces
- Frozen vegetables

FRUITS

The lowest G.I. fresh fruit choices include:

- Cherries
- Grapefruit
- Pears
- Apples
- Plums
- Peaches
- Oranges
- Grapes
- Kiwi
- Dried fruits, such as dried apricots, fruit medley, raisins, prunes etc.
- Canned peaches, pears, apple as a useful standby

DAIRY FOODS

- Shelf-stable skim milk or skim milk powder—easy to use in cooking
- Canned evaporated skim milk
- Cook 'n' Serve Sugar Free Pudding and Pie Filling

USEFUL FLAVORINGS, SAUCES AND DRESSINGS

- Spices—curry powder, cumin, turmeric, mustard etc.
- Herbs—oregano, basil, thyme etc.
- Bottled minced ginger, chili and garlic
- Sauces (such as soy, chili, oyster, hoi sin, teriyaki, Worcestershire)

- Bouillon
- Low oil salad dressings

WHAT TO KEEP IN THE REFRIGERATOR AND FREEZER

Dairy foods
- Skim or 1% milk
- Nonfat plain yogurt
- Light fruited yogurt
- Low fat ice cream
- Frozen low fat yogurt, sorbet, gelato
- Eggs

Cheese
- Low fat processed slices
- Reduced fat Swiss (such as Jarlsberg Light)
- Grated parmesan
- 1% or 2% cottage or part skim ricotta cheese

Vegetables and legumes
- Frozen peas, corn, spinach, carrots, and so on.

Fruit
- Frozen berries and melon balls

Chapter 14

EXERCISE: WE CAN'T LIVE WITHOUT IT

THE BENEFITS OF EXERCISE
HOW TO GET MOVING
8 WAYS TO MAKE EXERCISE WORK FOR YOU

No health-related reference book would be complete without a few words about exercise. The sad fact is, a multitude of changes in living habits now mean that in both work and recreation we're more sedentary. The result? As a nation, we're overweight! We just don't burn up enough calories to account for the amount of food we're eating.

■

TO LOSE WEIGHT YOU NEED TO EAT FEWER CALORIES AND BURN MORE CALORIES——AND THAT MEANS GETTING REGULAR EXERCISE AND LEADING A MORE ACTIVE LIFESTYLE.

■

THE BENEFITS OF EXERCISE

Most people could tell you at least one health benefit of exercise (reduces blood pressure, lowers the risk of heart disease, improves circulation, increases stamina, flexibility and strength), but the most motivating aspect of exercise is feeling so good about yourself for doing it.

Exercise speeds up our metabolic rate. By increasing our caloric expenditure, exercise helps to balance our sometimes excessive caloric intake from food.

More movement makes our muscles better at using fat as a source of fuel. By improving the way insulin works, exercise increases the amount of fat we burn.

A low G.I. diet has the same effect. Low G.I. foods reduce the amount of insulin we need, which makes fat easier to burn and harder to store. Since it's body fat that you want to get rid of when you lose weight, exercise in combination with a low G.I. diet makes a lot of sense!

HOW TO GET MOVING

Getting more exercise doesn't necessarily mean daily aerobics classes and jogging around the block (although this is great if you want to do it). What it *does* mean is moving more in everyday living. It's the day-to-day things we do—shopping, ironing, chasing kids, walking from the train station—where we spend the bulk of our energy. Since so much of our lifestyle is designed now to reduce our physical exertion, it's become very important to catch bursts of physical activity wherever we can, to increase our energy output. It may mean using the stairs instead of the elevator, taking a 10 minute walk at lunch time, trotting on a treadmill while you watch the news or talk on the telephone, walking to the grocery store to get the Sunday paper, hiding the remote control, parking a half-mile from work or taking the dog for a walk each night. Whatever it means, do it. Even housework burns calories!

HOW EXERCISE KEEPS YOU MOVING

The effect of exercise doesn't stop when you do. People who exercise have higher metabolic rates, so their bodies continue to burn more calories every minute, even when they're asleep!

Besides increasing the incidental activity you will also benefit from some planned aerobic activity, which causes you to breathe more heavily and makes your heart beat faster. Walking, cycling, swimming and stair climbing are just a few examples. You'll need to accumulate a total of at least 30 minutes of this type of activity 5 to 6 days a week.

Remember that reduction in body weight takes time. Even after you've made changes in your exercise habits, your weight may not be any different on the scales. This is particularly true in women, whose bodies tend to adapt to increased caloric expenditure.

Whatever it takes for you to burn more calories, do it. Try to regard movement as an opportunity to improve your physical well being—not as an inconvenience.

■

EXERCISE MAKES OUR MUSCLES BETTER AT USING FAT AS A SOURCE OF FUEL.

■

8 WAYS TO MAKE EXERCISE WORK FOR YOU

Your exercise routine will bring you lots of benefits if you can:

1. See how it benefits you.
2. Enjoy what you do.
3. Feel that you can do it fairly well.
4. Fit it in with your daily life.
5. Keep it inexpensive.
6. Make it accessible.
7. Stay safe while doing it.
8. Make it socially acceptable to your peers.

■

EXERCISE—TAKE IT REGULARLY, NOT SERIOUSLY.

■

Chapter 15

YOUR QUESTIONS ANSWERED

CAN PEOPLE WITH DIABETES EAT AS MUCH
SUGAR AS THEY WANT?

ARE NATURALLY OCCURRING SUGARS
BETTER THAN REFINED SUGARS?

IS SUGAR FATTENING?

AND MORE . . .

Can people with diabetes eat as much sugar as they want?

Not as much as they want, necessarily, but perhaps more than you think. Research shows that moderate consumption of refined sugar (about 8 teaspoons) a day doesn't compromise blood sugar control. This means you can choose foods which contain refined sugar or even use small amounts of table sugar. Try to spread your sugar budget over a variety of nutrient rich foods that sugar makes more palatable. Remember, sugar is concealed in many foods—a can of soft drink contains about 40 grams of sugar.

Most foods containing sugar do not raise blood sugar levels any more than most starchy foods.

Golden Grahams (G.I. 71) contain 39% sugar while Rice Chex (G.I. 89) contain very little sugar. Many foods with large amounts of sugar have G.I. values close to 60—lower than white bread.

Sugar can be a source of enjoyment and help you limit your intake of high fat foods, but the blood sugar response to a food is hard to predict. Use the tables in this book and your own blood sugar monitoring as a guide.

Are naturally occurring sugars better than refined sugars?

Naturally occurring sugars are those found in foods such as fruit, vegetables and milk. Refined sugars are concentrated sources of sugar such as table sugar, honey or molasses.

The rate of digestion and absorption of naturally occurring sugars is no different, on average, from that of refined sugars. There is wide variation within both food groups, depending on the food. For example, the glycemic index of fruits ranges from 22 for cherries to 72 for watermelon. Similarly, among the foods containing refined sugars, some have low G.I. values, while others have high G.I. numbers. The glycemic index of sweetened yogurt is only 33, while each Life Savers candy has a glycemic index of 70 (the same as some breads).

Some nutritionists argue that naturally occurring sugars are better because they contain minerals and vitamins not found in refined sugar. However, recent studies which have analyzed high sugar and low sugar diets clearly show that the diets overall contain similar amounts of micronutrients. Studies have shown that people who eat moderate amounts of refined sugars have perfectly adequate micronutrient intakes.

I've always heard that sugar is fattening. Is it?

No. Sugar has no special fattening properties—in fact, it is no more likely to be turned into fat than any other carbohydrate. Sugar, which you'll often find in foods high in calories and fat may sometimes seem to be "turned into fat," but it's the total number of calories you're consuming rather than the sugar in those calorie dense foods that may contribute to new stores of fat.

Has the glycemic index been tested in long-term studies?

At least 12 studies to date have looked at the glycemic index in the diet in relation to long-term diabetes control. Some of these studies have been five weeks long, others, including ours, up to three months. All but one showed a clear benefit in improving blood sugar levels. People with high blood lipids (cholesterol, triglycerides) showed improvements in this area as well.

Why are diets that disregard widely accepted nutritional guidelines so fashionable right now?

Several best-selling books have been published promoting high protein diets and generating a lot of publicity. They have been seized upon as a viable weight loss panacea. But the fact is: Diets that limit major food groups do not work over the long haul.

Chapter 16

HOW TO USE
THE G.I. TABLE

*T*he following table is an A to Z listing of the glycemic index values of commonly eaten foods in the United States and Canada. Approximately 300 different foods are listed, including some new values for foods tested only recently.

The glycemic index shown next to each food is the average for that food using glucose as the standard (i.e., glucose has a glycemic index of 100, with other foods rated accordingly). The average may represent the mean of 10 studies of that food worldwide or only 2 to 4 studies. In a few instances, American data are different from the rest of the world and we show that data rather than the average. Rice and oatmeal fall into this category.

To check on a food's glycemic index, simply look for it by name in the alphabetic list. You may also find it under a food type—fruit, cookies.

Included in the tables is the carbohydrate (CHO) and fat content of a sample serving of the food. This is to help you keep track of the amount of fat and carbohydrate in your diet. The sample serving is not the recommended serving—it is just an example of a serving. The glycemic index does not depend on your serving size because it is a ranking of the glycemic effect of foods using carbohydrate-equivalent portion sizes. You can eat more of a low G.I. food or less of a high G.I. food and achieve the same blood sugar levels.

Remember when you are choosing foods, the glycemic index isn't the only thing to consider. In terms of your blood sugar levels you should also consider the amount of carbohydrate you are eating. For your overall health the fat, fiber and micronutrient content of your diet is also important. A dietitian can guide you further with good food choices; see "For More Information" on page 103 for advice on finding a dietitian.

Chapter 17

THE GLYCEMIC INDEX TABLE

A–Z OF FOODS WITH GLYCEMIC INDEX, CARBOHYDRATE & FAT

Food	Glycemic Index	Fat (g per svg.)	CHO (g per svg.)
Agave nectar (90% fructose syrup), 1 tablespoon	11	0	16
All-Bran with extra fiber™, Kellogg's, breakfast cereal, ½ cup, 1 oz.	51 (av)	1	22
Angel food cake, ½ cake, 1 oz.	67	trace	17
Apple, 1 medium, 5 ozs.	38 (av)	0	18
Apple, dried, 1 oz.	29	0	24
Apple juice, unsweetened, 1 cup, 8 ozs.	40	0	29
Apple cinnamon muffin, from mix, 1 muffin	44	5	26
Apricots, fresh, 3 medium, 3 ozs.	57	0	12
canned, light syrup, 3 halves	64	0	14
dried, 5 halves	31	0	13
Apricot jam, no added sugar, 1 tablespoon	55	0	17
Apricot and honey muffin, low fat, from mix, 1 muffin	60	4	27
Bagel, 1 small, plain, 2.3 ozs.	72	1	38
Baked beans, ½ cup, 4 ozs.	48 (av)	1	24
Banana bread, 1 slice, 3 ozs.	47	7	46
Banana, raw, 1 medium, 5 ozs.	55 (av)	0	32
Banana, oat and honey muffin, low fat from mix, 1 muffin	65	4	27
Barley, pearled, boiled, ½ cup, 2.6 ozs.	25 (av)	0	22
Basmati white rice, boiled, 1 cup, 6 ozs.	58	0	50
Beets, canned, drained, ½ cup, 3 ozs.	64	0	5
Black bean soup, ½ cup, 4 ½ ozs.	64	2	19
Black beans, boiled, ¾ cup, 4.3 ozs.	30	1	31
Black bread, dark rye, 1 slice, 1.7 ozs.	76	1	18
Blackeyed peas, canned, ½ cup, 4 ozs.	42	1	16
Blueberry muffin, 1 muffin, 2 ozs.	59	4	27
Bran			
All-Bran with extra fiber™, Kellogg's, ½ cup, 1 oz.	51	1	20

Food	Glycemic Index	Fat (g per svg.)	CHO (g per svg.)
Bran Buds with Psyllium™, Kellogg's, ⅓ cup, 1 oz.	45	1	24
Bran Flakes, Post, ⅔ cup, 1 oz.	74	1	22
Multi-Bran Chex™, General Mills, 1 cup, 2.1 ozs.	58	1.5	49
Oat bran, 1 tablespoon	55	1	7
Oat bran muffin, 2 ozs.	60	4	28
Rice bran, 1 tablespoon	19	2	5
Breads			
Dark rye, Black bread, 1 slice, 1.7 ozs.	76	1	18
Dark rye, Schinkenbrot, 1 slice, 2 ozs.	86	1	22
French baguette, 1 oz.	95	1	15
Gluten-free bread, 1 slice	90	1	18
Hamburger bun, 1 prepacked bun, 1½ ozs.	61	2	22
Kaiser roll, 1, 2 ozs.	73	2	34
Light deli (American) rye, 1 slice, 1 oz.	68	1	16
Melba toast, 6 pieces, 1 oz.	70	2	23
Natural Ovens 100% Whole Grain, 1 slice, 1.2 ozs.	51	0	17
Natural Ovens Hunger Filler, 1 slice, 1.2 ozs.	59	0	16
Natural Ovens Natural Wheat, 1 slice, 1.2 ozs.	59	0	16
Natural Ovens Happiness, 1 slice, 1.1 oz.	63	0	15
Pita bread, whole wheat, 6½ inch loaf, 2 ozs.	57	2	35
Pumpernickel, whole grain, 1 slice, 1 oz.	51	1	15
Rye bread, 1 slice, 1 oz.	65	1	15
Sourdough, 1 slice, 1½ ozs.	52	1	20
Sourdough rye, Arnold's, 1 slice, 1½ ozs.	57	1	21
White, 1 slice, 1 oz.	70 (av)	1	12
100% stoneground whole wheat, 1 slice, 1½ ozs.	53	1	15
Whole wheat, 1 slice, 1 oz.	69 (av)	1	13
Bread stuffing from mix, 2 ozs.	74	5	13
Breakfast cereals			
All-Bran with extra fiber™, Kellogg's, ½ cup, 1 oz.	51	1	20
Bran Buds with Psyllium™, Kellogg's, ½ cup, 1 oz.	45	1	24
Bran Flakes, Post, ⅔ cup, 1 oz.	74	1	22
Cheerios™, General Mills, 1 cup, 1 oz.	74	2	23
Cocoa Krispies™, Kellogg's, 1 cup, 1 oz.	77	1	27
Corn Bran™, Quaker Crunchy, ¾ cup, 1 oz.	75	1	23
Corn Chex™, Nabisco, 1 cup, 1 oz.	83	0	26
Corn Flakes™, Kellogg's, 1 cup, 1 oz.	84 (av)	0	24
Cream of Wheat, instant, 1 packet, 1 oz.	74	0	21

Food	Glycemic Index	Fat (g per svg.)	CHO (g per svg.)
Cream of Wheat, old fashioned, ¾ cup, cooked, 6 ozs.	66	0	21
Crispix™, Kellogg's, 1 cup, 1 oz.	87	0	25
Frosted Flakes™, Kellogg's, ¾ cup, 1 oz.	55	0	28
Golden Grahams™, General Mills, ¾ cup, 1.6 ozs.	71	1	25
Grapenuts™, Post, ¼ cup, 1 oz.	67	1	27
Grapenuts Flakes™, Post, ¾ cup, 1 oz.	80	1	24
Life™, Quaker, ¾ cup, 1 oz.	66	1	25
Muesli, natural muesli, ⅔ cup, 1½ ozs.	56	3	28
Muesli, breakfast cereal, toasted, ⅔ cup, 2 ozs.	43	10	41
Multi-Bran Chex™, General Mills, 1 cup, 2.1 ozs.	58	1.5	49
Oat bran, raw, 1 tablespoon	55	1	7
Oat bran™, Quaker Oats, ¾ cup, 1 oz.	50	1	23
Oatmeal (made with water), old fashioned, cooked, ½ cup, 4 ozs.	49 (av)	1	12
Oats, 1-minute, Quaker Oats, 1 cup, cooked	66	2	25
Puffed Wheat™, Quaker, 2 cups, 1 oz.	67	0	22
Raisin Bran™, Kellogg's, ¾ cup, 1 oz.	73	0	32
Rice bran, 1 tablespoon	19	2	5
Rice Chex™, General Mills, 1¼ cups, 1 oz.	89	0	27
Rice Krispies™, Kellogg's, 1¼ cups, 1 oz.	82	0	26
Shredded wheat, spoonsize, ⅔ cup, 1.2 ozs.	58	0	27
Shredded Wheat™, Post, breakfast cereal 1 oz.	83	1	23
Smacks™, Kellogg's, ¾ cup, 1 oz.	56	1	24
Special K™, Kellogg's, 1 cup, 1 oz.	66	0	22
Team Flakes™, Nabisco, ¾ cup, 1 oz.	82	0	25
Total™, General Mills, ¾ cup, 1 oz.	76	1	24
Weetabix™, 2 biscuits, 1.2 ozs.	75	1	28
Buckwheat groats, cooked, ½ cup, 2.7 ozs.	54 (av)	1	20
Bulgur, cooked, ⅔ cup, 4 ozs.	48 (av)	0	23
Bun, hamburger, 1 prepacked bun, 1.7 ozs.	61	2	22
Butter beans, boiled, ½ cup, 4 ozs.	31 (av)	0	16
Cakes			
Angel food cake, 1 slice, 1⁄12 cake, 1 oz.	67	trace	17
Banana bread, 1 slice, 3 ozs.	47	7	46
Pound cake, homemade, 1 slice, 3 ozs.	54	15	42
Sponge cake, 1 slice, 1⁄12 cake, 2 ozs.	46	4	32
Capellini pasta, cooked, 1 cup, 6 ozs.	45	1	53
Cantaloupe, raw, ¼ small, 6½ ozs.	65	0	16

Food	Glycemic Index	Fat (g per svg.)	CHO (g per svg.)
Carrots, peeled, boiled, canned, ½ cup, 2.4 ozs.	49	0	3
Carrots, peeled, boiled, canned, ½ cup, 2.4 ozs.	49	0	3
Cereal grains			
Barley, pearled, boiled, ½ cup, 2.6 ozs.	25 (av)	0	22
Bulgur, cooked, ½ cup, 3 ozs.	48 (av)	0	17
Couscous, cooked, ½ cup, 3 ozs.	65 (av)	0	21
Corn			
Cornmeal, whole grain, from mix, cooked, ⅓ cup, 1.4 ozs.	68	1	30
Sweet corn, canned, drained, ½ cup, 3 ozs.	55 (av)	1	15
Taco shells, 2 shells, 1 oz.	68	5	17
Rice			
Basmati, white, boiled, 1 cup, 6 ozs.	58	0	50
Brown, 1 cup, 6 ozs.	55 (av)	0	37
Converted™, Uncle Ben's, 1 cup, 6 ozs.	44	0	38
Instant, cooked, 1 cup, 6 ozs.	87	0	37
Long grain, white, 1 cup, 6 ozs.	56 (av)	0	42
Parboiled, 1 cup, 6 ozs.	48	0	38
Rice cakes, plain, 3 cakes, 1 oz.	82	1	23
Short grain, white, 1 cup, 6 ozs.	72	0	42
Chana dal, ½ cup, 4 ozs.	8	3	28
Cheerios™, General Mills, breakfast cereal, 1 cup, 1 oz.	74	2	23
Cherries, 10 large cherries, 3 ozs.	22	0	10
Chickpeas (garbanzo beans), canned, drained, ½ cup, 4 ozs.	42	2	15
boiled, ½ cup, 3 ozs.	33 (av)	2	23
Chocolate butterscotch muffin, low fat from mix, 1 muffin	53	4	29
Chocolate, bar, 1½ ozs.	49	14	26
Chocolate Flavor, Nestle Quik™ (made with water), 3 teaspoons	53	0	14
Coca-Cola™, soft drink, 1 can	63	0	39
Cocoa Krispies™, Kellogg's, breakfast cereal, 1 cup, 1 oz.	77	1	27
Corn			
Cornmeal, cooked from mix, ⅓ cup, 1.4 ozs.	68	1	30
Sweet corn, canned and drained, ½ cup, 3 ozs.	55 (av)	1	15
Corn Bran™, Quaker Crunchy, breakfast cereal, ¾ cup, 1 oz.	75	1	23
Corn Chex™, General Mills, breakfast cereal, 1 cup, 1 oz.	83	0	26
Corn chips, 1 oz.	72	10	16
Corn Flakes™, Kellogg's, breakfast cereal, 1 cup, 1 oz.	84 (av)	0	24
Cornmeal, from mix, cooked, ⅓ cup, 1.4 ozs.	68	1	30

Food	Glycemic Index	Fat (g per svg.)	CHO (g per svg.)
Cookies			
Graham crackers, 4 squares, 1 oz.	74	3	22
Milk Arrowroot, 3 cookies, ½ oz.	69	2	9
Oatmeal, 1 cookie, ⅔ oz.	55	3	12
Shortbread, 4 small cookies, 1 oz.	64	7	19
Social Tea™ biscuits, Nabisco, 4 cookies, ⅔ oz.	55	3	13
Vanilla wafers, 7 cookies, 1 oz.	77	4	21
see also Crackers			
Couscous, cooked, ⅔ cup, 4 ozs.	65 (av)	0	21
Crackers			
Crispbread, 3 crackers, ⅔ oz.	81	0	15
Kavli™ All Natural Whole Grain Crispbread, 4 wafers, 1 oz.	71	1	16
Premium soda crackers, saltine, 8 crackers, 1 oz.	74	3	17
Rice cakes, plain, 3 cakes, 1 oz.	82	1	23
Ryvita™ Tasty Dark Rye Whole Grain Crisp Bread, 2 slices, ⅔ oz.	69	1	16
Stoned wheat thins, 3 crackers, ⅘ oz.	67	2	15
Water cracker, Carr's, 3 king size crackers, ⅘ oz.	78	2	18
Cream of Wheat, instant, 1 packet, 1 oz.	74	0	21
Cream of Wheat, old fashioned, ¾ cup, cooked, 6 ozs.	66	0	21
Crispix™, Kellogg's, breakfast cereal, 1 cup, 1 oz.	87	0	25
Croissant, medium, 1.2 ozs.	67	14	27
Custard, ½ cup, 4.4 ozs.	43	4	24
Dairy foods and nondairy substitutes			
Ice cream, 10% fat, vanilla, ½ cup, 2.2 ozs.	61 (av)	7	16
Ice milk, vanilla, ½ cup, 2.2 ozs.	50	3	15
Milk, whole, 1 cup, 8 ozs.	27 (av)	9	11
skim, 1 cup, 8 ozs.	32	0	12
chocolate flavored, 1%, 1 cup, 8 ozs.	34	3	26
Pudding, ½ cup, 4.4 ozs.	43	4	24
Soy milk, 1 cup, 8 ozs.	31	7	14
Tofu frozen dessert (nondairy), low fat, ½ cup, 2 ozs.	115	1	21
Yogurt			
nonfat, fruit flavored, with sugar, 8 ozs.	33	0	30
nonfat, plain, artificial sweetener, 8 ozs.	14	0	17
nonfat, fruit flavored, artificial sweetener, 8 ozs.	14	0	16
Dates, dried, 5, 1.4 ozs.	103	0	27
Doughnut with cinnamon and sugar, 1.6 ozs.	76	11	29
Fanta™, soft drink, 1 can	68	0	47

Food	Glycemic Index	Fat (g per svg.)	CHO (g per svg.)
Fava beans, frozen, boiled, ½ cup, 3 ozs.	79	0	17
Fettucine, cooked, 1 cup, 6 ozs.	32	1	57
Fish sticks, frozen, oven-cooked, fingers, 3½ ozs.	38	14	24
Flan cake, ½ cup, 4 ozs.	65	5	23
French baguette bread, 1 oz.	95	0	15
French fries, large, 4.3 ozs.	75	22	46
Frosted Flakes™, Kellogg's, breakfast cereal, ¾ cup, 1 oz.	55	0	28
Fructose, pure, 3 packets	23 (av)	0	10
Fruit cocktail, canned in natural juice, ½ cup, 4 ozs.	55	0	15
Fruits and fruit products			
Agave nectar (90% fructose syrup), 1 tablespoon	11	0	16
Apple, 1 medium, 5 ozs.	38 (av)	0	18
Apple, dried, 1 oz.	29	0	24
Apple juice, unsweetened, 1 cup, 8 ozs.	40	0	29
Apricots, fresh, 3 medium, 3.3 ozs.	57	0	12
canned, light syrup, 3 halves	64	0	19
dried, 1 oz.	31	0	13
Apricot jam, no added sugar, 1 tablespoon	55	0	17
Banana, raw, 1 medium, 5 ozs.	55 (av)	0	32
Cantaloupe, raw, ¼ small, 6½ ozs.	65	0	16
Cherries, 10 large, 3 ozs.	22	0	10
Dates, dried, 5, 1.4 ozs.	103	0	27
Fruit cocktail, canned in natural juice, ½ cup, 4 ozs.	55	0	15
Grapefruit, raw, ½ medium, 3.3 ozs.	25	0	5
Grapefruit juice, unsweetened, 1 cup, 8 ozs.	48	0	22
Grapes, green, 1 cup, 3 ozs.	46 (av)	0	15
Kiwi, 1 medium, raw, peeled, 2½ ozs.	52 (av)	0	8
Mango, 1 small, 5 ozs.	55 (av)	0	19
Marmalade, 1 tablespoon	48	0	17
Orange, navel, 1 medium, 4 ozs.	44 (av)	0	10
Orange juice, 1 cup, 8 ozs.	46	0	26
Papaya, ½ medium, 6½ ozs.	58 (av)	0	14
Peach, fresh, 1 medium, 3 ozs.	28	0	7
canned, natural juice, ½ cup, 4 ozs.	30	0	14
canned, light syrup, ½ cup, 4 ozs.	52	0	18
canned, heavy syrup, ½ cup, 4 ozs.	58	0	26
Pear, fresh, 1 medium, 5 ozs.	38 (av)	0	21
canned in pear juice, ½ cup, 4 ozs.	44	0	13

Food	Glycemic Index	Fat (g per svg.)	CHO (g per svg.)
Pineapple, fresh, 2 slices, 4 ozs.	66	0	10
Pineapple juice, unsweetened, canned, 8 ozs.	46	0	34
Plums, 1 medium, 2 ozs.	39 (av)	0	7
Raisins, ¼ cup, 1 oz.	64	0	28
Strawberry jam, 1 tablespoon	51	0	18
Watermelon, 1 cup, 5 ozs.	72	0	8
Gatorade™ sports drink, 1 cup, 8 ozs.	78	0	14
Glucose powder, 2½ tablets	102	0	10
Gluten-free bread, 1 slice, 1 oz.	90	1	18
Golden Grahams™, General Mills, ¾ cup, 1.6 ozs.	71	1	25
Granola Bars™, Quaker Chewy, 1 oz.	61	2	23
Gnocchi, cooked, 1 cup, 5 ozs.	68	3	71
Graham crackers, 4 squares, 1 oz.	74	3	22
Grapefruit, raw, ½ medium, 3.3 ozs.	25	0	5
Grapefruit juice unsweetened, 1 cup, 8 ozs.	48	0	22
Grapenuts™, Post, breakfast cereal, ¼ cup, 1 oz.	67	1	27
Grapenuts Flakes™, Post, breakfast cereal, ¾ cup, 1 oz.	80	1	24
Grapes, green, 1 cup, 3.3 ozs.	46 (av)	0	15
Green pea soup, canned, ready to serve, 1 cup, 9 ozs.	66	3	27
Hamburger bun, 1 prepacked bun, 1½ ozs.	61	2	22
Honey, 1 tablespoon	58	0	16
Ice cream, 10% fat, vanilla, ½ cup, 2.2 ozs.	61 (av)	7	16
Ice milk, vanilla, ½ cup, 2.2 ozs.	50	3	15
Isostar, 1 cup, 8 ozs.	73	0	18
Jelly beans, 10 large, 1 oz.	80	0	26
Kaiser rolls, 1 roll, 2 ozs.	73	2	34
Kavli™ All Natural Whole Grain Crispbread, 4 wafers, 1 oz.	71	1	16
Kidney beans, red, boiled, ½ cup, 3 ozs.	27 (av)	0	20
Kidney beans, red, canned and drained, ½ cup, 4.3 ozs.	52	0	19
Kiwi, 1 medium, raw, peeled, 2½ ozs.	52 (av)	0	8
Kudos Granola Bars™ (whole grain), 1 bar, 1 oz.	62	5	20
Lactose, pure, ⁷⁄₁₀ oz.	46 (av)	0	10
Lentil soup, Unico, canned, 1 cup, 8 ozs.	44	1	24
Lentils, green and brown, boiled, ½ cup, 3 ozs.	30 (av)	0	16
Lentils, red, boiled, 1.4 cup, 4 ozs.	26 (av)	0	27
Life™, Quaker, breakfast cereal, ¾ cup, 1 oz.	66	1	25
Life Savers™, roll candy, 6 pieces, peppermint	70	0	10
Light deli (American) rye bread, 1 slice, 1 oz.	68	1	16

FOOD	GLYCEMIC INDEX	FAT (G PER SVG.)	CHO (G PER SVG.)
Lima beans, baby, frozen, ½ cup, 3 ozs.	32	0	17
Linguine pasta, thick, cooked, 1 cup, 6 ozs.	46 (av)	1	56
Linguine pasta, thin, cooked, 1 cup, 6 ozs.	55 (av)	1	56
M&M's Chocolate Candies Peanut™, 1.7 oz. package	33	13	30
Macaroni and Cheese Dinner™, Kraft packaged, cooked, 1 cup, 7 ozs.	64	17	48
Macaroni, cooked, 1 cup, 6 ozs.	45	1	52
Maltose (maltodextrin), pure, 2½ teaspoons	105	0	10
Mango, 1 small, 5 ozs.	55 (av)	0	19
Marmalade, 1 tablespoon	48	0	17
Mars Almond Bar™, 1.8 ozs.	65	12	31
Melba toast, 6 pieces, 1 oz.	70	2	23
Milk, whole, 1 cup, 8 ozs.	27 (av)	9	11
skim, 1 cup, 8 ozs.	32	0	12
chocolate flavored, 1%, 1 cup, 8 ozs.	34	3	26
Milk Arrowroot, 3 cookies, ½ oz.	63	2	9
Millet, cooked, ½ cup, 4 ozs.	71	1	2
Muesli, breakfast cereal, toasted, ⅔ cup, 2 ozs.	43	10	41
Muesli, non-toasted, ⅔ cup, 1½ ozs.	56	3	28
Multi-Bran Chex™, General Mills, 1 cup, 2.1 ozs.	58	1.5	49
Muffins			
Apple cinnamon, from mix, 1 muffin, 2 ozs.	44	8	33
Apricot and honey, low fat, from mix, 1 muffin	60	4	27
Banana, oat and honey, low fat, from mix, 1 muffin	65	4	27
Blueberry, 1 muffin, 2 ozs.	59	4	27
Chocolate butterscotch, low fat, from mix, 1 muffin	53	4	29
Oat and raisin, low fat, from mix, 1 muffin	54	3	28
Oat bran, 1 muffin, 2 ozs.	60	4	28
Mung beans, boiled, ½ cup, 3½ ozs.	38	1	18
Natural Ovens 100% Whole Grain bread, 1 slice, 1.2 ozs.	51	0	17
Natural Ovens Hunger Filler bread, 1 slice, 1.2 ozs.	59	0	16
Natural Ovens Natural Wheat bread, 1 slice, 1.2 ozs.	59	0	16
Natural Ovens Happiness bread, 1 slice, 1.1 ozs.	63	0	15
Navy beans, boiled, ½ cup, 3 ozs.	38 (av)	0	
Nutella™ (spread), 2 tablespoons, 1 oz.	33	9	19
Oat and raisin muffin, low fat from mix, 1 muffin	54	3	28
Oat bran, 1 tablespoon	55	1	7

Food	Glycemic Index	Fat (g per svg.)	CHO (g per svg.)
Oat bran™, Quaker Oats, breakfast cereal, ¾ cup, 1 oz.	50	1	23
Oat bran, 1 muffin, 2 ozs.	60	4	28
Oatmeal (made with water), old fashioned, cooked, 1 cup, 8 ozs.	49	2	26
Oatmeal cookie, 1, ⅗ oz.	55	3	12
Oats, 1-minute, Quaker Oats, 1 cup, cooked	66	2	25
Orange, navel, 1 medium, 4 ozs.	44 (av)	0	10
Orange syrup, diluted, 1 cup	66	0	20
Orange juice, 1 cup, 8 ozs.	46	0	26
Papaya, ½ medium, 5 ozs.	58 (av)	0	14
Parsnips, boiled, ½ cup, 2½ ozs.	97	0	15
Pasta			
Capellini, cooked, 1 cup, 6 ozs.	45	1	53
Fettucine, cooked, 1 cup, 6 ozs.	32	1	57
Gnocchi, cooked, 1 cup, 5 ozs.	68	3	71
Linguine thick, cooked, 1 cup, 6 ozs.	46 (av)	1	56
Linguine thin, cooked, 1 cup, 6 ozs.	55 (av)	1	56
Macaroni, cooked, 1 cup, 5 ozs.	45	1	52
Macaroni & Cheese Dinner™, Kraft, packaged, cooked, 1 cup, 7 ozs.	64	17	48
Ravioli, meat-filled, cooked, 1 cup, 9 ozs.	39	8	32
Spaghetti, white, cooked, 1 cup, 6 ozs.	41 (av)	1	52
Spaghetti, whole wheat, cooked, 1 cup, 6 ozs.	37 (av)	1	48
Spirali, durum, cooked, 1 cup, 6 ozs.	43	1	56
Star Pastina, cooked, 1 cup, 6 ozs.	38	1	56
Tortellini, cheese, cooked, 8 ozs.	50	6	26
Vermicelli, cooked, 1 cup, 6 ozs.	35	0	42
Pastry, flaky, ⅛ of double crust, 2 ozs.	59	15	24
Pea soup, split with ham, canned, 1 cup, Wil-Pak Foods, 5½ ozs.	66	7	56
Peach, fresh, 1 medium, 3 ozs.	28	0	7
canned, heavy syrup, ½ cup, 4 ozs.	58	0	26
canned, light syrup, ½ cup, 4 ozs.	52	0	18
canned, natural juice, ½ cup, 4 ozs.	30	0	14
Peanuts, roasted, salted, ½ cup, 2½ ozs.	14 (av)	38	16
Pear, fresh, 1 medium, 5 ozs.	38 (av)	0	21
canned in pear juice, ½ cup, 4 ozs.	44	0	13
Peas, green, fresh, frozen, boiled, ½ cup, 2.7 ozs.	48 (av)	0	11
Peas dried, boiled, ½ cup, 2 ozs.	22	0	7

Food	Glycemic Index	Fat (g per svg.)	CHO (g per svg.)
Pineapple, fresh, 2 slices, 4 ozs.	66	0	10
Pineapple juice, unsweetened, canned, 8 ozs.	46	0	34
Pinto beans, canned, ½ cup, 4 ozs.	45	1	18
Pinto beans, soaked, boiled, ½ cup, 3 ozs.	39	0	22
Pita bread, whole wheat, 6½ inch loaf, 2 ozs.	57	2	35
Pizza, cheese and tomato, 2 slices, 8 ozs.	60	22	56
Plums, 1 medium, 2 ozs.	39 (av)	0	7
Popcorn, light, microwave, 2 cups (popped)	55	3	12
Potatoes			
Desirée, peeled, boiled, 1 medium, 4 ozs.	101	0	13
French fries, large, 4.3 ozs.	75	26	49
instant mashed potatoes, Carnation Foods™, ½ cup, 3½ ozs.	86	2	14
new, unpeeled, boiled, 5 small (cocktail), 6 ozs.	62 (av)	0	23
new, canned, drained, 5 small, 6 ozs.	61	0	23
red-skinned, peeled, boiled, 1 medium, 4 ozs.	88 (av)	0	15
red-skinned, baked in oven (no fat), 1 medium, 4 ozs.	93 (av)	0	15
red-skinned, mashed, ½ cup, 4 ozs.	91 (av)	0	16
red-skinned, microwaved, 1 medium, 4 ozs.	79	0	15
sweet potato, peeled, boiled, ½ cup mashed, 3 ozs.	54 (av)	0	20
white-skinned, peeled, boiled, 1 medium, 4 ozs.	63 (av)	0	24
white-skinned, with skin, baked in oven (no fat), 1 medium, 4 ozs.	85 (av)	0	30
white-skinned, mashed, ½ cup, 4 ozs.	70 (av)	0	20
white-skinned, with skin, microwaved, 1 medium, 4 ozs.	82	0	29
Sebago, peeled, boiled, 1 medium, 4 ozs.	87	0	13
Potato chips, plain, 14 pieces, 1 oz.	54 (av)	11	15
Pound cake, 1 slice, homemade, 3 ozs.	54	15	42
Power Bar™, Performance, Chocolate, 1 bar	58	2	45
Premium saltine crackers, 8 crackers, 1 oz.	74	3	17
Pretzels, 1 oz.	83	1	22
Puffed Wheat™, Quaker, breakfast cereal, 2 cups, 1 oz.	67	0	22
Pumpernickel bread, whole grain, 2 slices	51	2	30
Pumpkin, peeled, boiled, mashed, ½ cup, 4 ozs.	75	0	6
Raisins, ¼ cup, 1 oz.	64	0	28
Raisin Bran™, Kellogg's, breakfast cereal, ¾ cup, 1.3 ozs.	73	0	32
Ravioli, meat-filled, cooked, 1 cup, 9 ozs.	39	8	32
Rice			
Basmati, white, boiled, 1 cup, 7 ozs.	58	0	50

Food	Glycemic Index	Fat (g per svg.)	CHO (g per svg.)
Brown, 1 cup, 6 ozs.	55 (av)	0	37
Converted™, Uncle Ben's, 1 cup, 6 ozs.	44	0	38
Instant, cooked, 1 cup, 6 ozs.	87	0	37
Long grain, white, 1 cup, 6 ozs.	56 (av)	0	42
Parboiled, 1 cup, 6 ozs.	48	0	38
Rice bran, 1 tablespoon	19	2	5
Rice cakes, plain, 3 cakes, 1 oz.	82	1	23
Short grain, white, 1 cup, 6 ozs.	72	0	42
Rice Chex™, General Mills, breakfast cereal, 1¼ cups, 1 oz.	89	0	27
Rice Krispies™, Kellogg's, breakfast cereal, 1¼ cups, 1 oz.	82	0	26
Rice vermicelli, cooked, 6 ozs.	58	0	48
Roll (bread), Kaiser, 1 roll, 2 ozs.	73	2	39
Romano (cranberry) beans, boiled, ½ cup, 3 ozs.	46	0	21
Rutabaga, peeled, boiled, ½ cup, 2.6 ozs.	72	0	3
Rye bread, 1 slice, 1 oz.	65	1	15
Ryvita™ Tasty Dark Rye Whole Grain Crisp Bread, 2 slices, ⅔ oz.	69	1	16
Sausages, smoked link, pork and beef, fried, 2½ ozs.	28	29	5
Semolina, cooked, ⅔ cup, 6 ozs.	55	0	17
Shortbread, 4 small cookies, 1 oz.	64	7	19
Shredded Wheat™, Post, breakfast cereal, 1 oz.	83	1	23
Shredded wheat, 1 biscuit, ⅙ oz.	62	0	19
Skittles Original Fruit Bite Size Candies™, 2.3 oz. pk.	70	3	59
Smacks™, Kellogg's, breakfast cereal, ¾ cup, 1 oz.	56	1	24
Snickers™, 2.2 oz. bar	41	15	36
Social Tea™ biscuits, Nabisco, 4 cookies, ⅔ oz.	55	3	13
Soft drink, Fanta™, 1 can, 12 ozs.	68	0	47
Soups			
Black bean soup, ½ cup, 4½ ozs.	64	2	19
Green pea soup, canned, ready to serve, 1 cup, 9 ozs.	66	3	27
Lentil soup, Unico, canned, 1 cup, 8 ozs.	44	1	24
Pea soup, split, with ham, Wil-Pak Foods, 1 cup, 5½ ozs.	66	7	56
Tomato soup, canned, 1 cup, 9 ozs.	38	4	33
Sourdough bread, 1 slice, 1½ ozs.	52	1	20
Rye bread, Arnold's, 1 slice, 1½ ozs.	57	1	21
Soy beans, boiled, ½ cup, 3 ozs.	18 (av)	7	10
Soy milk, 1 cup, 8 ozs.	31	7	14
Spaghetti, white, cooked, 1 cup	41 (av)	1	52
Spaghetti, whole wheat, cooked, 1 cup, 5 ozs.	37 (av)	1	48

Food	Glycemic Index	Fat (g per svg.)	CHO (g per svg.)
Special K™, Kellogg's, breakfast cereal, 1 cup, 1 oz.	66	0	22
Spirali, durum, cooked, 1 cup, 6 ozs.	43	1	56
Split pea soup, 8 ozs.	60	4	38
Split peas, yellow, boiled, ½ cup, 3½ ozs.	32	0	21
Sponge cake plain, 1 slice, 3 ½ ozs.	46	4	32
Sports drinks			
Gatorade™ 1 cup, 8 ozs.	78	0	14
Isostar, 1 cup, 8 ozs.	73	0	18
Sportsplus, 1 cup, 8 ozs.	74	0	17
Sports bars			
Power Bar™, Performance Chocolate Bar, 1 bar	58	2	45
Stoned wheat thins, 3 crackers, ⅙ oz.	67	2	15
Strawberry Nestle Quik™ (made with water), 3 teaspoons	64	0	14
Strawberry jam, 1 tablespoon	51	0	18
Sucrose, 1 teaspoon	65 (av)	0	4
Syrup, fruit flavored, diluted, 1 cup	66	0	20
Sweet corn, canned, drained, ½ cup, 3 ozs.	55 (av)	1	16
Sweet potato, peeled, boiled, ½ cup mashed, 3 ozs.	54 (av)	0	20
Taco shells, 2 shells, 1 oz.	68	5	17
Tapioca pudding, boiled with whole milk, 1 cup, 10 ozs.	81	13	51
Taro, peeled, boiled, ½ cup, 2 ozs.	54	0	23
Team Flakes™, Nabisco, breakfast cereal, ¾ cup, 1 oz.	82	0	25
Tofu frozen dessert, nondairy, low fat, 2 ozs.	115	1	21
Tomato soup, canned, 1 cup, 9 ozs.	38	4	33
Tortellini, cheese, cooked, 8 ozs.	50	6	26
Total™, General Mills, breakfast cereal, ¾ cup, 1 oz.	76	1	24
Twix Chocolate Caramel Cookie™, 2, 2 ozs.	44	14	37
Vanilla wafers, 7 cookies, 1 oz.	77	4	21
Vermicelli, cooked, 1 cup, 6 ozs.	35	0	42
Vitasoy™ Soy milk, creamy original, 1 cup, 8 ozs.	31	7	14
Waffles, plain, frozen, 4 inch square, 1 oz.	76	3	13
Water crackers, 3 king size crackers, ⅙ oz.	78	2	18
Watermelon, 1 cup, 5 ozs.	72	0	8
Weetabix™ breakfast cereal, 2 biscuits, 1.2 ozs.	75	1	28
White bread, 1 slice, 1 oz.	70 (av)	1	12
Whole wheat bread, 1 slice, 1 oz.	69 (av)	1	13
Yam, boiled, 3 ozs.	51	0	31

Food	Glycemic Index	Fat (g per svg.)	CHO (g per svg.)
Yogurt			
nonfat, fruit flavored, with sugar, 8 ozs.	33	0	30
nonfat, plain, artificial sweetener, 8 ozs.	14	0	17
nonfat, fruit flavored, artificial sweetener, 8 ozs.	14	0	16

GLYCEMIC INDEX TESTING

If you are a food manufacturer, you may be interested in having the glycemic index of some of your products tested on a fee-for-service basis. For more information, contact either:

Glycaemic Index Testing Inc.
135 Mavety Street
Toronto, Ontario
Canada M6P 2L8
E-mail: thomas.wolever@utoronto.ca

or

Sydney University Glycaemic Index Research Service (SUGIRS)
Department of Biochemistry
University of Sydney
NSW 2006 Australia
Fax: (61)(2) 9351-6022
E-mail: j.brandmiller@staff.usyd.edu.au

FOR MORE INFORMATION

REGISTERED DIETITIANS

Registered Dietitians (R.D.s) are nutrition experts who provide nutritional assessment and guidance and support. Check for the initials "RD" after the name to identify qualified dietitians who provide the highest standard of care to their clients. Glycemic index is part of their training so all dietitians should be able to help in applying the principles in this guide, but some dietitians do specialize in certain areas. If you want more detailed advice on glycemic index just ask the dietitian whether this is a specialty when you make your appointment.

Dietitians work in hospitals and often run their own private practices, as well. For a list of dietitians in your area, contact the American Dietetic Association (ADA) Consumer Nutrition Hotline (1-800-366-1655) or visit ADA's home page at the address below. You can also check the Yellow Pages under "Dietitians."

The American Dietetic Association
216 West Jackson Boulevard
Chicago, IL 60606
Phone: 1-800-877-1600
Fax: 1-312-899-1979
Web site: http://www.eatright.org/

SUGAR INFORMATION

The Sugar Association
1101 15th Street, NW, Suite 600
Washington, DC 20005
Web site: http://www.sugar.org

PRIMARY CARE PHYSICIANS

It's always a good idea to discuss any health problems or concerns with your primary care physician.

NATURAL OVENS ORDERING INFORMATION

Natural Ovens of Manitowoc
4300 County Trunk CR
P.O. Box 730
Manitowoc WI 54221-0730
Telephone: 1-800-772-0730
Fax: 920-758-2594
http://www.naturalovens.com/

ACKNOWLEDGMENTS

We would like to acknowledge the extraordinary efforts of Johanna Burani and Linda Rao, who adapted this book—and the other books in *The Glucose Revolution Pocket Guide* series—for North American readers. Together they have worked to ensure that every piece of information is accurate and appropriate for readers in the U.S. and Canada.

For more information about *The Glucose Revolution* and *The Glucose Revolution Pocket Guides*, visit **www.glucoserevolution.com**

ABOUT THE AUTHORS

Kaye Foster-Powell, B.Sc., M. Nutr. & Diet., is an accredited dietitian-nutritionist in both public and private practice in New South Wales, Australia. A graduate of the University of Sydney (B.Sc., 1987; Master of Nutrition and Dietetics, 1994), she has extensive experience in diabetes management and has researched practical applications of the glycemic index over the last five years. A co-author of *The Glucose Revolution* and all the titles in *The Glucose Revolution Pocket Guide* Series, she lives in Sydney, Australia.

Jennie Brand-Miller, Ph.D., Associate Professor of Human Nutrition in the Human Nutrition Unit, Department of Biochemistry, University of Sydney, Australia, is widely recognized as one of the world's leading authorities on the glycemic index. She received her B.Sc. (1975) and Ph.D. (1979) degrees from the Department of Food Science and Technology at the University of New South Wales, Australia. She is the editor of the *Proceedings of the Nutrition Society of Australia* and a member of the Scientific Consultative Committee of the Australian Nutrition Foundation. She has written more than 200 research papers, including 60 on the glycemic index of foods. A co-author of *The Glucose*

Revolution and all the titles in *The Glucose Revolution Pocket Guide* Series, she lives in Sydney, Australia.

Thomas M.S. Wolever, M.D., Ph.D., another of the world's leading researchers of the glycemic index, is Professor in the Department of Nutritional Sciences, University of Toronto, and a member of the Division of Endocrinology and Metabolism, St. Michael's Hospital, Toronto. He is a graduate of Oxford University (B.A., M.A., M.B., B.Ch., M.Sc., and D.M.) in the United Kingdom. He received his Ph.D. at the University of Toronto. His research since 1980 has focused on the glycemic index of foods and the prevention of type 2 diabetes. A co-author of *The Glucose Revolution* and all the titles in *The Glucose Revolution Pocket Guide* Series, he lives in Toronto, Canada.

Johanna Burani, M.S., R.D., C.D.E., is a registered dietitian and certified diabetes educator with more than 10 years experience in nutritional counseling. She specializes in designing individual meal plans based on low glycemic-index food choices. The adapter of *The Glucose Revolution* and co-adapter, with Linda Rao, of all the titles in *The Glucose Revolution Pocket Guide* Series, she is the author of seven books and professional manuals, and lives in Mendham, New Jersey.

Linda Rao, M.Ed., a freelance writer and editor, has been writing and researching health topics for the past 11 years. Her work has appeared in several national publications, including *Prevention* and *USA Today*. She serves as a contributing editor for *Prevention* Magazine and is the co-adapter, with Johanna Burani, of all the titles in *The Glucose Revolution Pocket Guide* Series. She lives in Allentown, Pennsylvania.

The Glucose Revolution begins here . . .

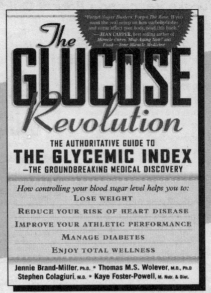

THE GLUCOSE REVOLUTION
THE AUTHORITATIVE GUIDE TO THE GLYCEMIC INDEX—
THE GROUNDBREAKING MEDICAL DISCOVERY

NATIONAL BESTSELLER!

"Forget *Sugar Busters.* Forget *The Zone.* If you want the real scoop on how carbohydrates and sugar affect your body, read this book by the world's leading researchers on the subject. It's the authoritative, last word on choosing foods to control your blood sugar."

—JEAN CARPER, best-selling author of *Miracle Brain, Miracle Cures, Stop Aging Now!* and *Food—Your Miracle Medicine*

ISBN 1-56924-660-2 • $14.95

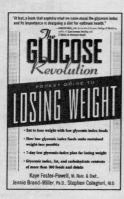
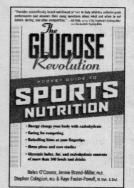

The Glucose Revolution Pocket Guide to
DIABETES

Help control your diabetes with low glycemic index foods

Based on the most up-to-date information about carbohydrates, this basic guide to the glycemic index and diabetes allows people with type 1 and type 2 diabetes to make more informed choices about their diets. Topics covered include why many traditionally "taboo" foods don't cause the unfavorable effects on blood sugar levels they were believed to have, and why diets based on low G.I. foods improve blood sugar control. Also covered are how to include more of the right kinds of carbohydrates in your diet, the

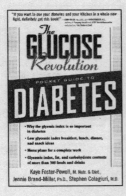

optimum diet for people with diabetes, practical hints for meal preparation and tips to help make the glycemic index work throughout the day, a week of low G.I. menus, G.I. success stories, and more.

ISBN 1-56924-675-0 • $4.95

The Glucose Revolution Pocket Guide to
YOUR HEART

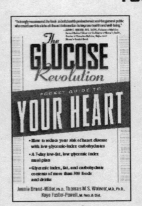

Healthy eating you can feel in your heart

The latest medical research clearly confirms that slowly digested low G.I. carbohydrates like pasta, grainy breads, cereals based on wheat bran and oats, and many popular Mediterranean-style foods play an important part in treating and preventing heart disease—in addition to controlling blood sugar and aiding weight loss. With 21 pages of charts, this handy pocket guide shows you how to choose the right amount of the right carbohydrates for reducing the risk of heart attack and for lifelong health and wellbeing.

ISBN 1-56924-640-8 • $4.95

THE TOP 100 LOW GLYCEMIC FOODS

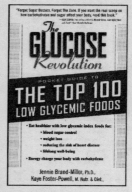

ISBN 1-56924-678-5 • $4.95

The best of the best in low glycemic index foods

The slow digestion and gradual rise and fall in blood sugar levels after a food with a low glycemic index has benefits for many people. Today we know the glycemic index of hundreds of different generic and name-brand foods, which have been tested following a standardized method. Now *The Top 100 Low Glycemic Foods* makes it easy to enjoy those slowly digested carbohydrates every day for better blood sugar control, weight loss, a healthy heart, and peak athletic performance.